pilates & golf

CW00758654

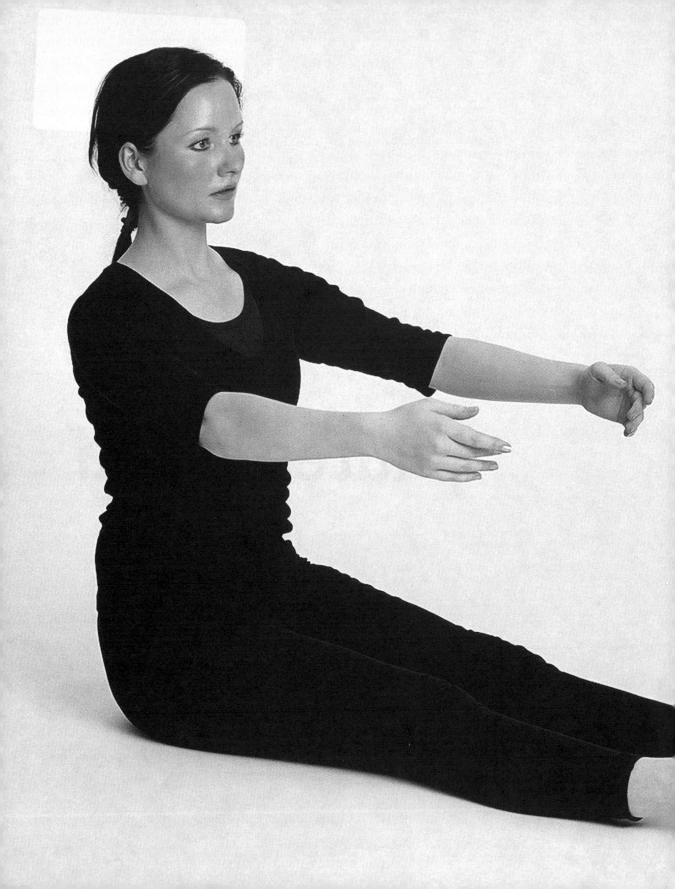

pilates & golf

MICHAEL KING

& NUALA COOMBS

PILATES & GOLF

by Michael King and Nuala Coombs

First published in Great Britain in 2005 by
Steedman Publishers Limited
Suite 8, 68 Broadwick Street, London W1F 9QZ

© Steedman Publishers Limited 2005

All rights reserved. No part of this publication may be reproduced or utilised in any form
by any means, electronic or mechanical, including photocopying, recording or by any
information storage and retrieval system, without prior permission of the publishers.

ISBN: 0-9550027-0-2

A CIP catalogue record for this book is available from the British Library.

While all reasonable care has been taken during the preparation of this edition, neither
the publisher, editors, nor the authors can accept responsibility for any consequences
arising from the use thereof or from the information contained therein.

Set in Bliss

Printed and bound by Hobbs the Printers Ltd, Totton, Hants.

Contents

ABOUT THE AUTHORS

Michael King

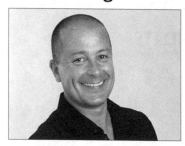

Michael King has been a fitness expert, educating and training people in the many facets of the fitness industry, since 1979.

Michael's formal dance training was with the London School of Contemporary Dance. He began integrating his dance training with his fitness career as a Pilates instructor and adult exercise instructor at the Pineapple Dance Studio in London before touring with the London Bach Festival throughout Europe.

Michael moved to Texas, joining the faculty at the Houston Ballet whilst also directing the Adult Fitness Programme and Pilates Studio. During his eight years with the Houston Ballet, Michael worked on numerous prestigious productions including the Nutcracker, Swan Lake, The Sleeping Beauty and Daphnis

and Chloe. Next – Los Angeles, where Michael taught for five years at the Voight Fitness and Dance Studio and was a personal trainer with an extensive celebrity client list. From L.A., he moved to Switzerland where he directed two health centres whilst continuing to travel world-wide.

Having been a teacher of Pilates for 22 years, Michael now works from his studio and training centre in the City, London. With the Pilates Institute team, he is the training provider for Pilates in many of the national fitness chains in the UK and around the world. He is also actively involved in developing the UK standards of education for the Pilates technique.

Michael's choreography of the world-acclaimed production of The Official Tribute to the Blues Brothers has been performed extensively both in the UK and Europe. With further projects such as My Fair Lady in Buenos Aires and Godspell in the UK, he continues to be an international name in the world of dance.

Nuala Coombs

Nuala has been involved in the fitness industry since 1979. Starting with the launch of her health club in 1979, she has taught all aspects of health and fitness since that time.

Nuala's technique expanded when she discovered Pilates in 1985 as a client and began to apply the principles she was learning to her teaching protocol.

As a Director of the Pilates Institute, she has been instrumental in the development of courses and delivers all aspects of the Pilates Institute Method both in the UK and abroad. She has also been involved in the development of Pilates' education standards in the UK.

Her extensive teaching background and varied expertise allows Nuala to present an open and varied approach to the Pilates technique.

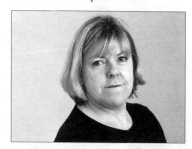

the pilates institute method

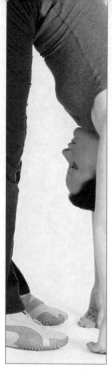

The pilates institute method

Throughout the years many Pilates studios have opened, teaching clients on an individual basis and also in groups as well as training instructors to teach the technique.

Each studio developed its own interpretation of the technique and over the years passed the skills down from teacher to teacher.

The original Pilates Method, taught by Joseph Pilates, is a unique and special technique that promotes flexibility, strength and coordination. However, he based the development of the training on his own physical abilities and those of the professional dancers who were the majority of his students. The studios were few and small, so clients were given very individual attention.

Today, with the popularity of group matwork classes and even group Pilates equipment sessions, the technique has naturally evolved into something quite different from the original concept.

The clients we are working with at the Pilates Institute often spend many hours at desks using computers or have a sedentary lifestyle. Cars, chairs and footwear also often affect posture. In addition, we have people starting the technique later in life whose flexibility and strength may need attention.

Although both the authors of this book were originally trained in the traditional Method, when research became available to us from physiotherapists in Australia carrying out research into low back pain, it became very clear that applying this evidence to our training style made sense. We felt it was only correct to take advantage of research that was not available in Joseph Pilates' day

The Pilates Institute programme is thus research and evidence based. Our background in fitness together with our Pilates training enables us to adapt the technique with an open approach. As a result, the basic training that we offer to newcomers to the Pilates technique is quite different from the traditional style.

The fundamental difference between the Pilates Institute Method and the traditional style is that the latter works with an imprinted spine and raises the head and shoulders off the floor for many of the movements, whereas the Pilates Institute Method works with a neutral spinal alignment and keeps the head and shoulders on the floor.

The effect of lifting the head

and shoulders from the floor is that the superficial abdominal muscles may become dominant in the movements. These muscles do not act as stabilisers for the spine and consequently it is possible that the muscles needed to allow safe and effective functional movement do not get targeted, so over time they do not function as well as they might. Of course these superficial muscles need to be exercised, but it is important that before they are activated, the deep stabilising muscles close to the spine are set, ready to support it whilst the larger muscles take care of movement.

The Pilates Institute Method starts at base level, educating the postural muscles to enable the various abdominal muscles to do their job effectively. Leaving the head and shoulders on the floor whilst learning how to perform the movements allows the client to focus on the connection and activation of the deep stabilising muscles needed to support the lumbar spine in particular. Once this body awareness is in place, the challenge becomes about maintaining good form whilst

performing the movements. The results are then significant. When these support muscles function well, the benefits of the Pilates Institute Method show through with quality of movement and improved technique.

Our wish for all our clients is that they work towards performing well the traditional style of Pilates as originally intended. However, it is important that they address posture issues first to avoid injury.

The Pilates Institute Method, allows participants to develop their abilities with the technique at their own pace and also takes into consideration individual needs by modifying the moves as necessary.

If this is your first introduction to the Pilates Institute Method either as someone experienced with or new to the Pilates Method, the opening chapters are very important. The fundamentals of the Pilates Institute Method are explained in detail. We recommend you familiarise yourself fully with the set up sequence before moving on to the repertoire and programmes.

Now there is nothing left to say but to encourage you to start learning about this great movement technique or to add to your existing skills.

Good luck ...

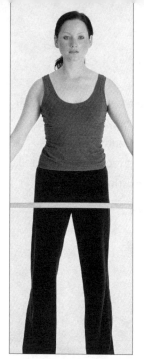

The pilates institute method and golf

Your body is the key to improving your golf swing and consequently your game. Today the Pilates technique is used widely within sports applications to enhance athletic technique. Many professional golfers have been using Pilates as a rehabilitation tool or as a preventative measure. It is this innovative approach to golf that has now put the focus on Pilates.

The game of golf requires a mind and body approach. Concentration, strength, flexibility and power are essential. The workload put on the spine and supporting structures is immense, and when the body is out of balance, the risk of injury intensifies. So logic leads us to conclude that if we work on muscular balance and alignment then we are not only reducing the risk of injury but also improving our game.

Many hours are spent working on improving the swing but problems are often the consequence of poor biomechanics.

The Pilates Institute Method will teach you how to get the best game available to you by helping you improve your postural stability, mobilise and strengthen your body where you need to in order to improve coordination, maximise your distance and add power to your game.

Be patient. Years of repetitive behaviour will take time to unravel. Practicing the Pilates Institute Method regularly will enable you to improve your body awareness and change movement patterns that may be affecting your game.

Start gradually and ensure you understand the basics before moving on to the more complicated programmes. With regular practice you will begin to notice improvements you didn't think possible.

Enjoy ...

THE HISTORY OF GOLF

The most popular theory about the origins of golf suggests we owe it all to a pastime of fishermen on the east coast of Scotland during the 15th century.

After mooring their boats, these fishermen would use pieces of driftwood to shoot small rocks across the rolling fields and sand dunes that marked their path home.

Whatever its origins the game caught on. So much so that during the mid-15th century, when Scotland was preparing for an invasion from England, King James II banned it. He felt the soldiers were too distracted by the game and were neglecting their military exercises.

The ban didn't stop ardent players, though. The Scots were so addicted to the game that they continued to play in secret. It wasn't until 1502 that King James IV, who took up the game himself, finally lifted the ban.

With this kind of royal endorsement, golf's popularity quickly spread throughout 16th century Europe. King Charles I brought the game to England

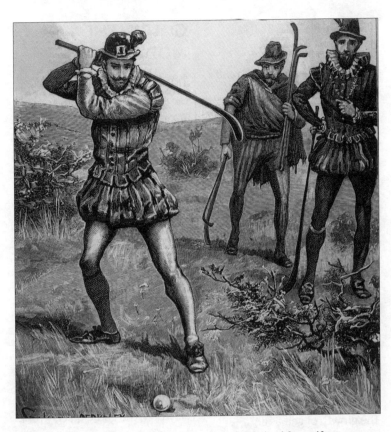

and Mary Queen of Scots introduced it to France. In fact, the term 'caddie' stems from the name she gave her attendants, known as cadets.

Despite its popularity with European royalty, it took 150 years before golf was organised into an official game. By the 17th century, a universally accepted body of rules was established.

Stroke play was introduced in 1759, and an 18-hole course was built in 1764 in Leith, Scotland. Eighteen holes became the de

facto standard for golf courses after that.

Also by this time, equipment had changed considerably from mere sticks and stones.

Club heads were made from beech or fruitwood. Some club heads were even made from hand-forged iron. Shafts were usually ash or hazel. Balls were made from boiled, tightly compressed goose feathers that were then wrapped in leather.

Very few people could afford such handcrafted equipment, and the game quickly earned a reputation as a rich man's pastime.

However, once metal clubs and rubber balls were invented by the mid 19th century, golf became affordable for the average person and its popularity soared. Golf associations and clubs began to form all over the UK. Small, local groups of enthusiasts who gathered to socialise, eat and drink formed the majority of clubs. In fact, the early clubs were more about kicking back with a jug of claret than playing golf. This might explain why the Open Championship trophy today is a claret jug!

The growth of golf as an organised, competitive sport in the UK was matched around the world, especially in Europe, India, Canada and America. This led to the first international golf tournament – the Amateur Golf Championship of India and the East in 1893.

By 1900 there were more than 1,000 golf clubs in North America alone. This was also the year that golf was made an Olympic sport, confirming its status as truly a world sport.

GOLF IN THE MODERN AGE

The dawn of the 20th century brought with it several technological innovations that changed the game of golf forever.

The first was the Haskell one-piece rubber cored ball, which virtually guaranteed an extra 20 yards. Grooved-faced irons were introduced in 1902. In 1905, the first dimpled ball was invented. Steel-shafted clubs came in 1910. Within the span of a decade, golfers could hit further and more accurately than ever before.

However, the game quickly took a back seat in Europe during the war years. The hiatus allowed the game to develop in virtual isolation in the US, and it was during this time that American golfers surged forward.

They built new and more challenging courses. They changed the rules, and introduced a larger ball that measured 1.66 inches in diameter. This required a different stroke but made for greater control of the ball.

Following World War II, golf gained even greater international exposure with the emergence of players such as Arnold Palmer, Gary Player and Jack Nicklaus. They propelled golf's popularity into the stratosphere and firmly entrenched the game in modern popular culture.

Today, players like Tiger Woods, and Mike Weir in the UK, have taken the game to new heights.

Yet throughout golf's history, one thing has remained the same. The essence of the game we know today is still very much the same as it was when a bunch of rambunctious fishermen pushed a couple of rocks around with driftwood on Scotland's rolling greens and sandy shores.

WHY THE PILATES INSTITUTE METHOD? AND WHY NOW?

Golf has become one of the most played recreational sports in the world over the past 10 years and has recently seen an explosion in popularity. Because it allows players of varying skill and ability to play and even compete, it has a large participant base.

A general misunderstanding about golf is that it does not require great physical ability. It is a sport that appears not to require separate fitness training to achieve a level of competence. This misconception leads to increased injury among beginners while more experienced players often play with existing and recurrent injuries. The most common areas of injury for the professional player are the wrist and hand (Batt, 1992). The spine is the second next most injured area for the professional and the most common area injured for the amateur (Batt, 1992) (Ibid).

The effect of the golf swing on an unstable spine is huge. The rotation and side bending that

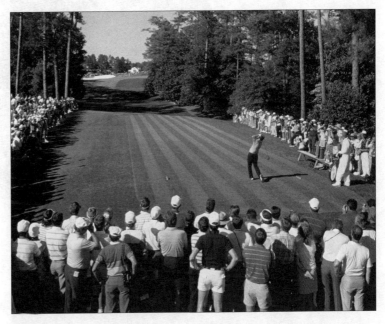

are necessary during its performance can cause excessive stress on structures of the spine.

The Pilates Institute Method will address these particular issues. The benefit of a Pilates Institute programme is the flexibility it gives you. You do not need expensive equipment and you will have the information to create your own effective pre-game warm up and strengthening programme. The Pilates Institute Method will allow the amateur as well as the professional to develop effective alignment and movement throughout the swing.

This programme will create a

strong and efficient group of postural muscles and when you learn how to engage them for optimum stability, will improve flexibility and power.

To improve the game we must study the following:

- Focus
- Posture
- Breathing
- Balance
- Core strength
- Flexibility for maximal range of movement – especially in shoulder and hip joints

The Pilates Institute Method will benefit all the above areas.

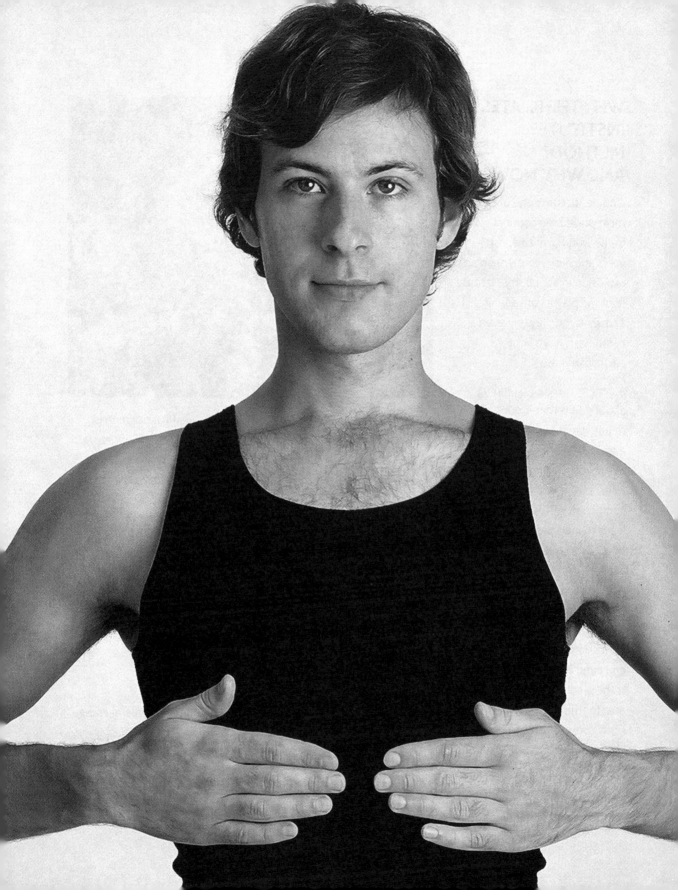

MODERN FITNESS TRENDS AND GOLF

Recently the fitness industry has been promoting the benefits of functional training and how an effective programme will improve our daily lives – but what is it?

The latest research on exercise encourages exercises that stimulate the central nervous system (CNS). Exercises that challenge balance and coordination and work with varying resistance loads help to improve the function of our CNS. The benefit of this is improved quality of life for daily activities.

The nervous system gathers information from our senses and perception of life around us. It processes this information and makes decisions for appropriate responses (movement).

When playing golf, for instance, we take in information about our surroundings – wind factor, terrain, etc. – and decide on our shot: whether we play a swing, chip or putt. The quality of the movement depends on the quality of the information being received. When we have a well balanced, stable posture and the information flow is good, then the quality of movement will be the best available.

It is generally agreed by fitness professionals and scientists alike that exercises that use multiple muscle groups and are applicable to physical tasks we perform during our daily lives are most beneficial. This means having the ability to balance and be coordinated whilst moving muscles and joints through various ranges of motion. Exercise equipment manufacturers are beginning to accept that isolating muscle groups by sitting the user in a set position may not get the best overall results. Stability and support from our back, arms and legs must come from our ability to control the muscles involved throughout a movement or exercise. To do this effectively we must learn to use our stabilising muscles.

Balance, coordination and flowing movement are all vital factors when we set about improving our golf game. The Pilates Institute Method effectively educates the body to take on these tasks. During any particular movement you will learn to control the muscles targeted whilst maintaining proper postural alignment with optimal stability of the torso.

The deep postural muscles used to develop a functional approach to your "Pilates for golf programme" are often referred to as the "core" or inner unit. These muscles are very close to the spine and are instrumental in stabilising the lumbar spine (lower back) when functioning well.

While you may have a strong and appealing-looking "six pack", these superficial abdominal muscles will not help to improve your game in the same way that learning to connect with your postural muscles will.

The goal of the Pilates Institute Method "Pilates for golf programme" is to teach you to recognise when you have optimal postural stability and maximise your potential for the perfect shot.

SO – WHAT IS THE CORE?

When we explain the "core" to clients, we compare it to a tree trunk. The closer to the centre one gets, the stronger the tree. The bark on the outside of the tree is like our superficial abdominal muscles, the ones we most commonly train. These large muscles are referred to as "global". They are close to the surface and are what we feel when we practice our standard abdominal exercises. A regular crunch is performed using the rectus abdominus, a sheet of muscle that runs down the front of our body and is known for creating the six-pack we work towards. This muscle flexes the spine forward but does little to stabilise it. Just like the tree, as we move closer to the centre of the body, we find the muscles responsible for support, particularly of the lumbar spine. This group of muscles are the deepest layer of abdominal muscles and closest to the spine. They are referred to as "local" muscles. All muscles work in synergy, but if we only focus on the superficial muscles such as rectus abdominus and ignore the core muscles necessary for support, then just

like a hollowed out tree with no centre to protect against the elements, our internal structure will be left vulnerable and open to injury.

To understand the importance of core stability in relation to exercise and sport we need to take a look at the anatomy of our "core" muscles, or "inner unit" as we refer to them throughout this book.

Our inner unit is made up like a cylinder. The top is the diaphragm, the sides are the corset of muscle known as the transversus abdominis (TA), the base is the pelvic floor and weaving through the back is the multifidus.

DIAPHRAGM – The diaphragm is a major muscle involved in respiration. It also increases the pressure inside the abdominal cavity, which contributes to spinal support.

TRANSVERSUS ABDOMINIS – This is the deepest of the abdominal muscles. Its actions are to draw in the abdominal wall and support the contents. It does not move the spine, but there is evidence that it assists

with spinal stability.

PELVIC FLOOR – The lower part (floor) of the pelvis is made up of layers of muscles and tissue that stretch like a hammock from the tail bone at the back to the pubic bone at the front. These muscles control the bladder and the bowels.

MULTIFIDUS – This deep muscle weaves from the base of the spine to the base of the neck. It helps to stabilise the lumbar spine and rotates the head.

When the muscles of this cylinder are functioning as a unit, the intra-abdominal pressure created helps to stabilise the lumbar spine.

Learning how to correctly initiate engagement of these stabilising muscles whilst carrying out exercise, sport or everyday activities will improve posture and performance. Postural stability will help develop a consistent swing plane.

pilates – the history

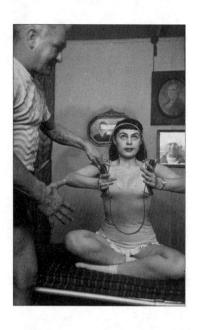

Pilates – the history

Joseph Hubertus Pilates was born in Germany in 1880. Although he was a frail child, suffering from asthma, rickets and rheumatic fever, he overcame his physical limitations with exercise and body-building. He became an accomplished gymnast, and upon leaving school joined the circus. At this time he was also teaching boxing. He moved to England in 1912, where he worked as a self-defence instructor with the UK police force.

At the outbreak of the First World War, Joseph Pilates was interned because he was a "German National" along with many other German nationals. He encouraged his fellow internees to exercise and put them through his regime.

Interestingly, there was very little illness in the camp where they were following his plan, unlike other camps where there had been fatalities due to an influenza epidemic. Word spread about this man and his exercise technique, and he was moved into a hospital as a medical aide. He couldn't stand by watching patients lying in bed wasting away, so he attached springs to the head of the beds and began

a programme of resistance training with the springs acting as tension. The result was that patients who were exercising recovered more quickly.

At the end of the war Joseph Pilates returned to Germany, but after a brief spell there training the German police force and the newly reorganized German army, he left for America.

On the ship to New York, Joseph Pilates met his wife Clara and on arrival they opened an exercise studio where he started teaching his technique. Martha Graham, who was also exploring new ways of movement and was considered a revolutionary in the dance world at that time,

encouraged her company to attend Pilate's studio. Later, she would not be so positive. The stories tell of strong personalities clashing. This did not, however, affect the popularity of Pilates' technique. It quickly became a favourite with dancers, who have used it through the years not only to strengthen their bodies but also to rehabilitate after injury. Joseph Pilates didn't dance himself, but the people around him obviously influenced his teachings. In video footage of social gatherings with Joseph Pilates, there are always dancers in his company.

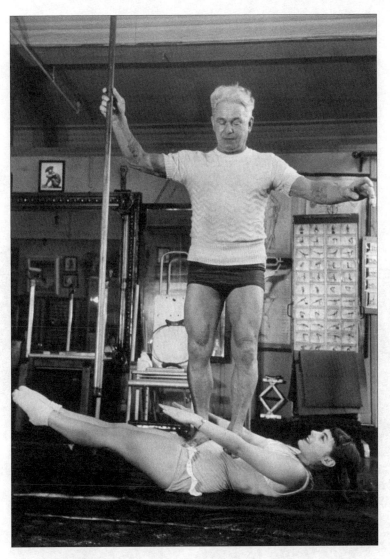

Modifications to the original technique now take into account those participants who may not be as strong, flexible and fit as Joseph Pilates was, but who can nevertheless benefit enormously from the technique.

Today more than ever, applying Joseph Pilates' principles to your exercise regime can only enhance and refine it. He referred to his programme as one that utilised mind, body and spirit, elements that are still equally important today.

Golf is a mind/body activity that requires finesse and control in order to achieve high standards. Applying the principles of Pilates to your game will inevitably create the focus and concentration needed to improve your physical and mental approach, resulting in a more pleasurable experience, reduced risk of injury and improved performance.

We will always acknowledge the dedication and hard work Joseph Pilates put into developing his corrective exercise Method.

Since his death in 1967, his technique has been subject to interpretation by many training schools. He did not specifically train anyone to present his work. Although his wife Clara continued to educate students and instructors in the Method, there was no formal school. This has resulted in a diverse and creative expression of his work, and many influential instructors have successfully continued to follow his basic principles.

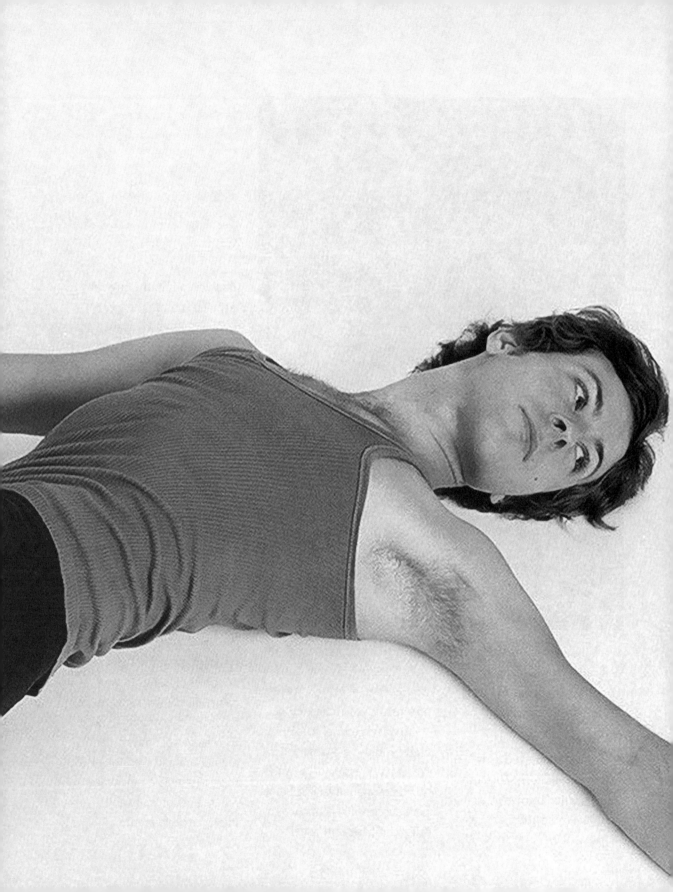

the principles

Introduction to the principles

These principles are the underpinning philosophy for the quality and performance of Pilates exercises. Joseph Pilates was very keen that the performance of the movements should be carried out with excellent form. Keeping his principles in mind will help you achieve this high standard.

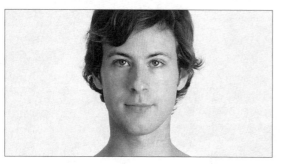

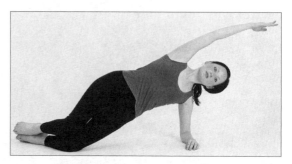

CONCENTRATION

"It is the mind that shapes the body"
(Joseph Pilates)

Concentration is the key to any mind/body programme. In order to train the motor skills required to carry out the Pilates Institute Method, you will need a peaceful place in which to practice, free from distraction. You will need to concentrate fully and focus your mind on the exact performance of the movements, gradually improving your ability to re-create the best possible quality of movement available to you at any given time. This ability to re-create movement patterns is essential to the development of your golf game.

CONTROL

Pilates movements are executed with control; nothing is haphazard. The Pilates Institute Method teaches slow, precise movements in order to facilitate focus on all the principles being in place. This element of the Pilates principles is exactly what is required in golf training. The golf swing needs control and strength. Without these, technique suffers. It is important to understand that the principles work in synergy, each one enhancing the other.

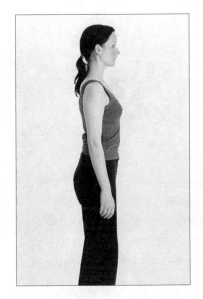

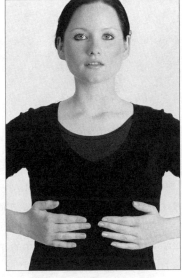

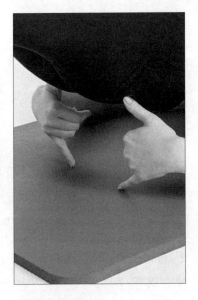

CENTRING

What Joseph Pilates called the powerhouse is what we refer to today as the core. Although we now have much more information available to us regarding body mechanics, the concept is the same. Working from a strong centre to stabilise our extremities essentially creates the same result whether we use an unstable surface to force a reaction or we teach ourselves to use our trunk muscles efficiently. Without a strong centre, our body is less effective and more vulnerable to injury. A strong core and postural stability will allow the golfer to maintain the spine angle throughout the swing.

BREATHING

Coordinated, conscious lateral patterns of breathing initiate movements and help to maintain the consistent mild contraction required for the Pilates Institute Method. This focus will also assist with the control of movement.

PRECISION

Joseph Pilates was very keen to establish precise quality of movement at each session. It is this conscious practice to ensure exact repetition of movement quality that is important, not the intensity or number of repetitions carried out.

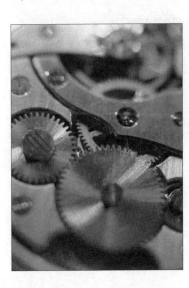

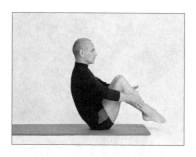 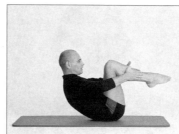 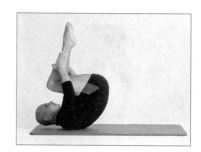

FLOWING MOVEMENT

Pilates is often compared to Tai Chi. The flowing movement is just what we aim to achieve with our Pilates practice. When we are learning, the movements are gradual and progressive in order to establish focus, concentration and the mind/body connection. As we become more proficient, our ability to sustain quality and create a continuous flow of movement becomes more natural. This combination of quality and precision is also beneficial to a great game of golf.

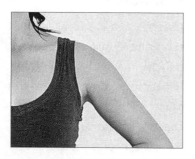

ISOLATION

In order to bring together all elements of the Pilates technique, the ability to isolate particular areas of the body and focus on stabilising and mobilising as best we can is an essential skill. This increased body awareness will manifest itself in an improved golf game.

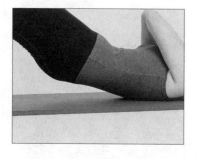

ROUTINE

Practice, practice, practise is the key to improvement in all things. The ability to recreate precision and quality of movement is a skill all serious sports people want to master. In Pilates, just as in golf, routine is an essential principle.

"Patience and persistence are vital qualities in the ultimate successful accomplishment of any worthwhile endeavour."
(Joseph Pilates)

the importance of good posture and golf

the importance of good posture and golf

"...incorrect stance and faulty posture greatly affect the success of the entire swing."
(Hogan, 1985)

POSTURE

Definition: the relative position or attitude of the body at any one period of time. Correct posture is the position when minimal stress is applied to the joints.

Not many golfers consider how their posture affects their overall game. Not only does correct posture improve your swing, it also eases the strain on your back, reducing the potential for injury.

Correct posture may seem an easy skill to master. Standing with knees flexed, back straight and bending from the hips shouldn't be that difficult,. However, muscular imbalance, stiffness and lack of stability brought about by our jobs, lifestyle and previous injuries can seriously affect our ability to achieve a good set up.

The set up is the most important aspect of the

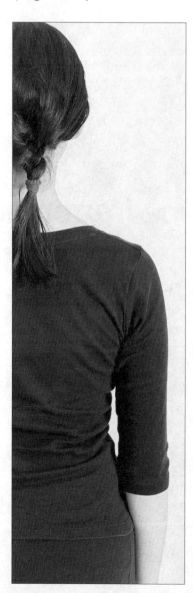

mechanics of the swing. Without this firm foundation you have little chance of a good result. The set up also affects the stresses and strains placed on the body throughout the swing phase. Attention to this detail is important if your game is to move on.

Good set up and foot positioning will allow you to maintain your balance throughout and create power and control. A good set up gives you an advantage from the start.

The posture you bring to your golf game has not just arrived with you at the club house. Your posture has been developing since you were born and will take time and concentrated effort to change.

Consider how many times you swing your golf club during a lifetime. If you don't try to correct faulty alignment, over time the consequences could be extremely painful, without considering the effect it will have on your game.

Faulty movement patterns and muscular imbalances may appear gradually over time, or if you are new to the game may be aggravated by the repetitious nature of play. Here are some common problems associated with muscular imbalances:

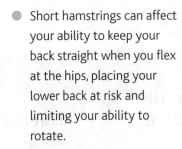

- Short hamstrings can affect your ability to keep your back straight when you flex at the hips, placing your lower back at risk and limiting your ability to rotate.

- Reduced range of motion in the hips will compromise your swing.

- Tension in the neck and shoulders will reduce your range of motion in neck rotation, causing discomfort and inability to follow the ball.

- Slumped posture from weak trunk and postural muscles will compress the trunk and reduce the range of motion and power. This posture will affect your depth of breath, which will also have a generally debilitating effect on your game.

- Inability to correctly stabilise the shoulders will increase the risk of injury.

These imbalances will have a cumulative effect, in that compensations will occur to allow the body to adapt to the gradual changes occurring in posture.

The Pilates Institute Method will teach you to stabilise the spine and the muscles that support it, which in turn will improve your posture, swing power and accuracy.

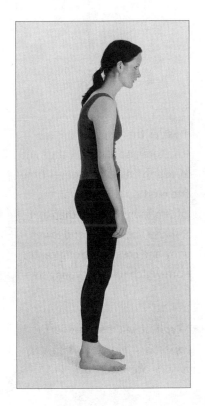

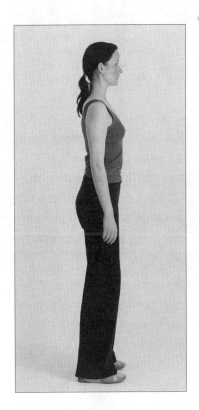

CONSIDER YOUR POSTURE

Four types of postural alignment

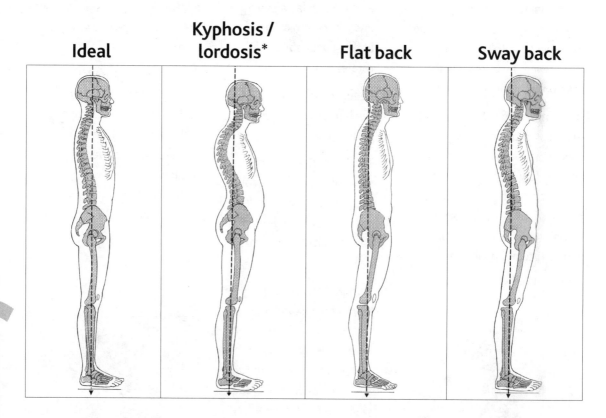

| Ideal | Kyphosis / lordosis* | Flat back | Sway back |

Just like the perfect swing, there is no such thing as perfect posture. Your foundation posture will almost certainly affect how you address the set up, perform your swing and ultimately play your game of golf.

The pictures above show the most common postures that we see. None of them is life threatening, but they are the result of imbalances brought about by strong short muscles and weak long muscles creating change in the natural curves of the spine. Any change in shape in any of the curves in the spine will create compensation throughout. Any instability in the shoulder girdle or pelvic girdle will alter posture, and the effect can ripple through the whole body from the feet to the top of the head.

The Pilates Institute Method focuses on the deep postural muscles that support this structure and allows change and re-alignment to occur over time. The Method will give you the information to strengthen and stabilise your upper and lower body and create a strong centre from which to focus your game.

Kyphosis is a roundness in the upper back and lordosis is a deep curve in the lower back.

It is apparent from the chart on the right that the stance addressed in golf places stress on the spine, particularly spinal flexion.

The lumbar spine is the most commonly injured area of the body for the amateur golfer (Batt, 1992). The swing, even if it is performed perfectly, places excessive stresses on the spine. Even professional players with their highly developed fitness and ability will suffer. In 1990, 24% of the professionals on the Professional Golfers' Association of America (PGA) tour had some form of lower back pain (McCarrol & Gioe).

Strength and stability of the deep abdominal and lower back muscles are necessary to control the rotational movement involved in the swing.

Knee injuries are common, especially with an aging population participating in the sport. Existing problems such as arthritis and operations to knees can be adversely affected. The ability to stabilise the lower body becomes a necessity.

The hip is an important area of the body when playing golf. The pelvis links the upper to the

How different positions put different stress on our spine

Posture	% disc pressure
Lying prone	25
Side lying	75
Standing	100
Seated upright	140
Standing – 45 degree hip flexion	150
Seated – spinal flexion	185
Standing hip flexed, holding weight downward	220
Seated – forward flexed, holding weight downward	275

lower body. The external rotation required in the swing creates stresses, and any golf exercise programme should address hip mobility as well as stability.

The shoulders are also important when golf is the sport of choice. The Pilates Institute Method will specifically focus on shoulder stability.

The above is a very brief look at common injuries associated with playing golf. The answer is correct posture, alignment and stability to prevent them occurring. The player must be able to maintain balance and coordination throughout various ranges of movement

and negotiate rotation of the upper and lower body. The Pilates Institute Method is the key.

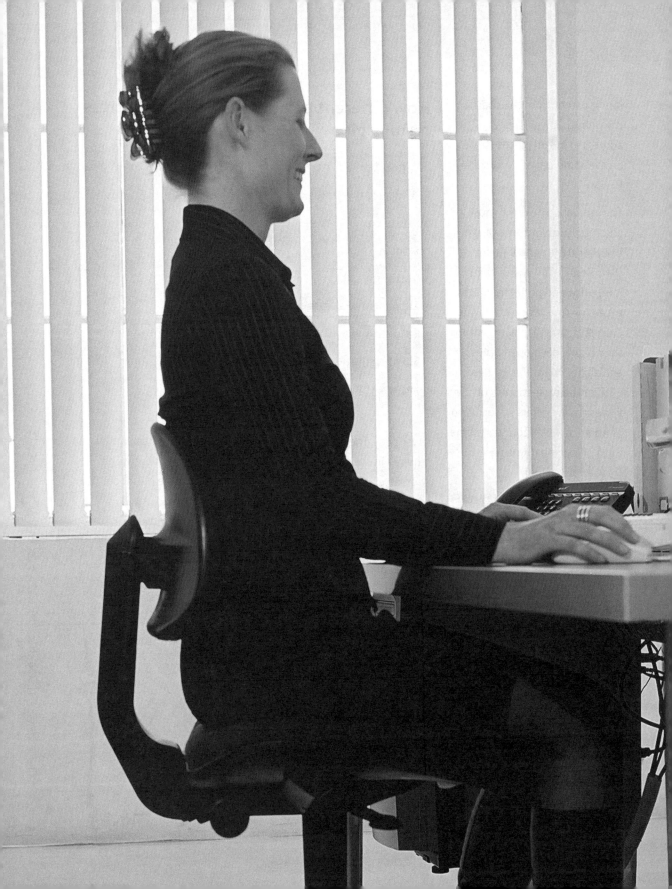

POSTURE IS POWER

Changing your posture can change your game

A great golf player needs consistency and accuracy when playing – having a good day can become less of a gamble than you think.

Improving your posture will definitely improve your swing. And as you train your postural muscles to work efficiently, this will show itself in the address and the performance of your swing and enable you to play consistently throughout the round.

However, to improve your posture you need to take a look at your lifestyle as a whole and not just when you play your round of golf.

How you use your body for everyday living will have just as much significance with regard to your posture as your game.

The position of your car seat, and the way you organise your work space or carry heavy packages or children, must be addressed. Just putting the Pilates Institute Method into practice for your game will not maintain the changes occurring.

A consistent mindfulness to your posture is needed.

Consider what you do on a daily basis that will affect your posture:

- Do you regularly drive for long periods of time?

- Does your job require you to stand/sit in one posture or carry out repetitive movements?

- Do you use a computer?

- Are your work surfaces correctly positioned for your height?

- Do you regularly wear stiletto heels (ladies!)

As you can see, there are many things not obviously connected to golf that will affect your posture, and of course you will take these imbalances onto the golf course. Whatever we do on a day-to-day basis affects our posture.

Applying the Pilates Institute Method not only to your game but to your everyday activities will gradually bring about the change you need to alleviate the effects of structural imbalances created by just living.

Remember though, your posture took time to develop and so will unravelling the knots. The key is consistency.

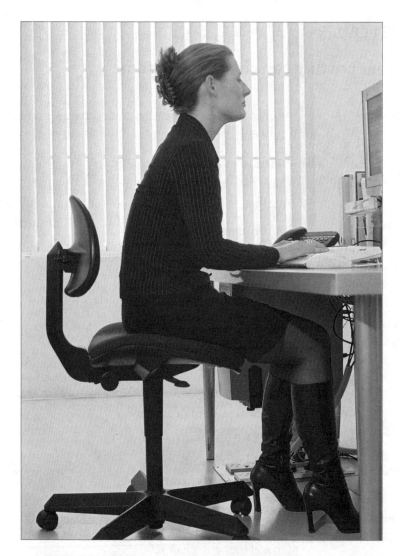

ARE YOU SITTING COMFORTABLY?

Then you are probably slouching. We are all guilty of this. The longer we sit in one position, the more likely we are to relax into our comfortable position – the one we don't have to think about but that, unfortunately, usually means we are causing stress to our spine.

Poor posture whilst working at a desk can cause headaches, tension and neck pain. To address these issues, check out your work station.

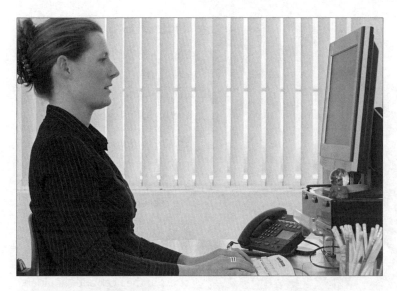

THE MONITOR

This should be at eye level – you should only need to move your eyes to see the complete screen. Use a monitor stand to bring your machine to the correct height. You can improvise with sturdy books. The monitor should also be placed directly in front of you, not off to the right or left, which will twist the spine and cause discomfort.

THE KEYBOARD

The keyboard should be straight in front of you. Try to keep your wrists straight. There are many wrist supports available at specialist shops that will help you maintain a good position.

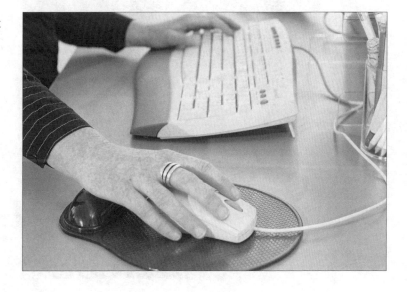

THE MOUSE

Keep your mouse close. Your arm should be parallel to the desk with your elbow a little lower. Try not to let the weight of your arm rest on the underside of your wrist. Again, a wrist support will help.

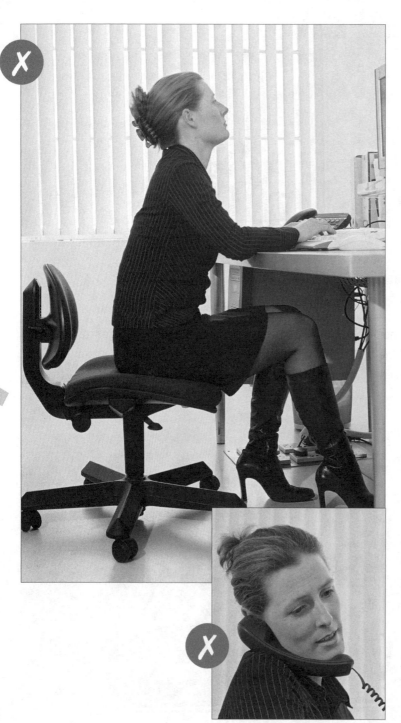

THE DESK

Your desk should be about navel height. You may need to raise your desk or alternatively, if it is too high, raise your chair.

Ensure that everything you need is within easy reach. When you use the telephone, don't hold the receiver between your ear and shoulder as you type. Continuously adopting this posture will create tension and stress in the neck and shoulders.

THE CHAIR

Ensure the chair is the correct height for you and the desk. Sit right back using the support provided by the seat, don't perch on the front. Draw your chair close to the desk so that you can easily reach the keyboard.

Sit with your hips slightly higher than your knees. If your chair doesn't have sufficient adjustment facilities, then use a wedge cushion to raise the hips at the back of the seat.

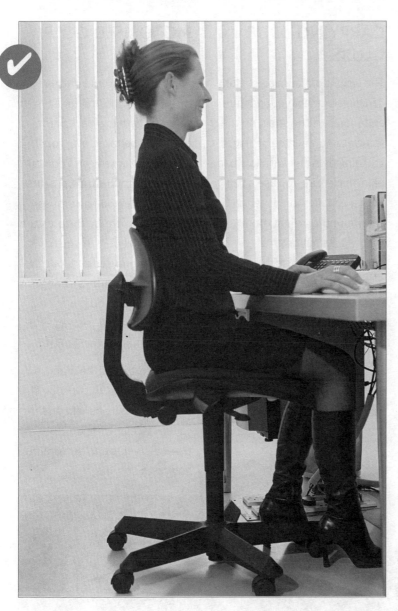

MOVING AROUND

Try to get up and walk about at least once an hour, change your position whilst sitting to reduce the potential for fatigue and think about using a stability ball instead of a chair for at least part of the day. The stability ball will force you to use your postural muscles, and the irresistible urge to bounce up and down on it will also reduce the onset of tiredness.

When you have taken the time to set up your work station, take a seat and try it on for size. Placing markers in relevant areas will help you maintain a good posture whilst you are sitting at your desk. A coloured dot (you can buy them at any stationers) where you know your correct eye line should be will remind you to sit up when you fall below the line. It is simple but effective.

Of course we cannot ignore the golf-specific postural pitfalls.

THE IMPORTANCE OF GOOD POSTURE AND GOLF

PUSHING OR PULLING YOUR CLUBS

Simply by pushing instead of pulling your golf trolley you can greatly reduce potential strain on the lower back. Pushing the trolley will enable you to keep it close to your body and avoid the side tracking that occurs when you pull the trolley behind you. If your course is hilly, however, then when going down hill it is safer to have the trolley behind you.

CARRYING YOUR CLUBS

The weight of your bag of clubs can hugely affect your posture and therefore the strain on the spine as you walk the course. If you already suffer with low back pain, make sure you use a bag with a double shoulder strap to distribute the weight more evenly. Take out any unnecessary load, such as clubs you never use. Use your "inner unit" to support your lower back by maintaining a mild contraction in as neutral a spine position as you can manage.

MOTORISED GOLF CARTS

Although one would imagine this would be helpful for anyone suffering with low back pain, care must be taken over rough terrain. Motorised carts do not promote a good sitting posture and the potential for surprise bumps will increase the pressure on the spinal discs. If you have to use a motorised cart, opt for the driving seat. The steering wheel will help you maintain a good posture and you can choose the smoothest path.

Of course, two of the main benefits of walking the course are the warm up benefit and the cardiovascular exertion. Both of these elements are lost when driving the course.

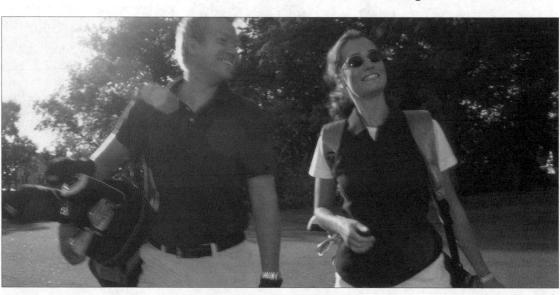

BENDING DOWN

Always remember that even the everyday action of bending over to pick something up has its hazards if not performed with mindfulness.

On the course you will bend over to pick up your golf ball many times. Remember:

- Use a split stance with one foot in front of the other – this will more evenly distribute the weight

- Engage that inner unit to support the lumbar spine

- If you need to, use your golf club to help support you

- Always bend your knees and hips. Avoid bending from the waist with straight legs.

In any situation where you need to bend, lean or pick something up – whether you are retrieving your ball on the golf course, picking up a package or child or even pushing a baby carriage – employ a correct, stabilising posture.

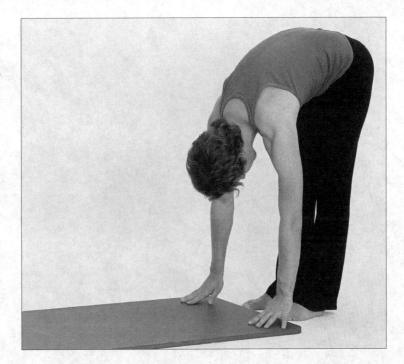

- Take a neutral pelvic position

- Engage your postural muscles to support and stabilise the lumbar spine

- Keep good shoulder alignment by allowing the shoulder blades to ease down the back

- Keep whatever you are lifting close to your body

- Ensure the height of the object you are pushing is correct and doesn't force you to lean at too great an angle, creating strain on the lower back

- Use a smooth and controlled motion.

Good posture and balance work together to produce a good shot. If you mix poor posture with poor balance, there is a hugely increased potential for bad play and injury.

The aim of the Pilates Institute Method in relation to your game of golf is to improve your balance whilst you are still and also during movement to allow you to stabilise your pelvis and shoulder girdle during your swing.

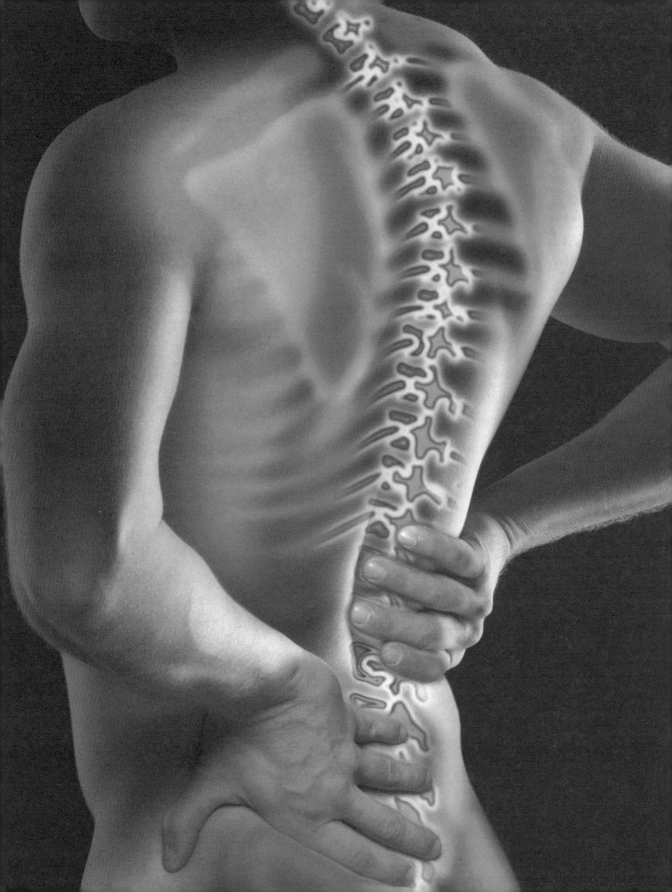

the pilates institute
programme for golf

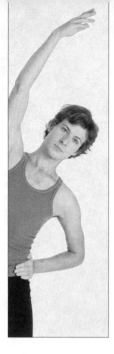

The pilates institute programme for golf

The basis of the Pilates Institute programme is the set up of the spine, the deep abdominal muscles and the breathing pattern.

- Spine in neutral alignment

- Mild contraction of the deep abdominals

- Lateral breath

FINDING YOUR NEUTRAL SPINAL ALIGNMENT

Lying on the floor, notice the natural shape of your lower back

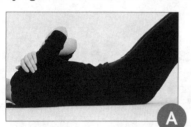

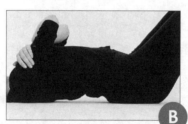

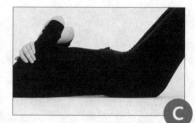

Gently roll your lower back into the floor, eliminating any natural curve (A)

Now roll your lower back in the opposite direction, creating an arch (B)

Now find the position half-way between these two points. This is your neutral spinal position (C)

This neutral spinal alignment is the starting point for all exercises in the programme. It may take some time to become a natural position for you, but it will become so with practice.

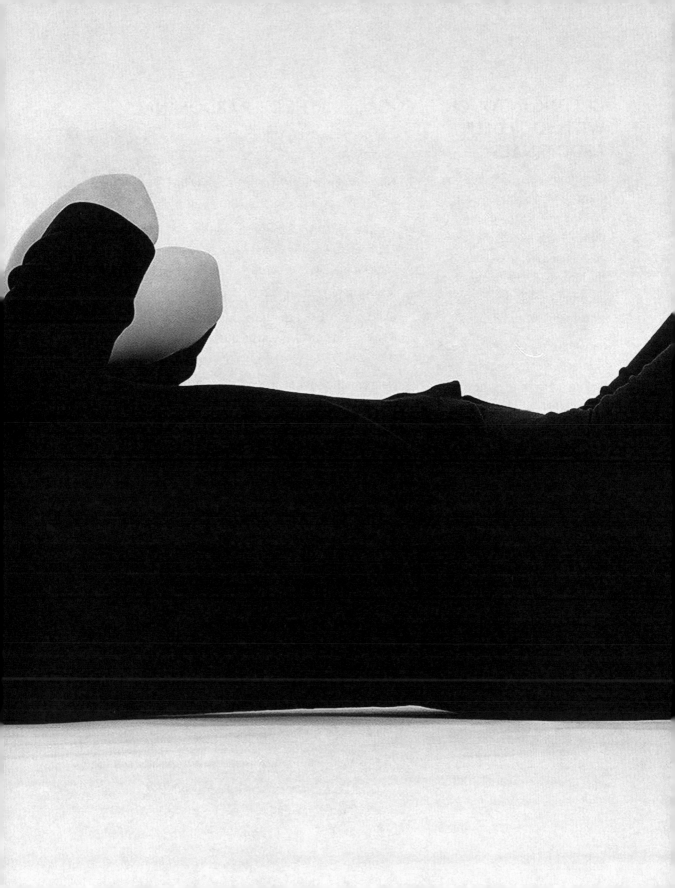

GETTING IN TOUCH WITH YOUR DEEP ABDOMINALS

Once you have established your neutral spinal alignment, you need to activate the muscles that will help to hold the posture and create stability in the lower back: the transversus abdominis, pelvic floor, diaphragm and multifidus.

Research has proved that a mild contraction of these deep abdominal muscles is the most effective way to allow a consistent contraction to be held for long periods of time because of the low load. It is important to know that the neutral spinal alignment and the mild contraction work together to create the potential for the optimal stability in the lower back that is essential for an effective swing.

ENGAGING THE DEEP ABDOMINALS

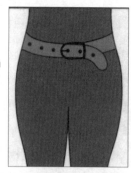

- First put yourself in neutral spine alignment.
- Now imagine you are wearing a belt with 10 notches on it.
- Breathe out and pull the belt in to the 10th notch. Breathe in and release the belt completely.

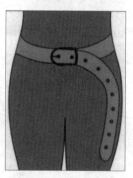

- Breathe out again and draw the belt in to the 10th notch but this time only release it to the 5th notch. As you breathe in, release.
- Next breathe out as you draw the belt to the 10th notch, release to the 5th notch and then just a tiny amount to the 3rd notch on the belt. This is the level of contraction required.
- Finally, release completely and then draw the belt straight to the 3rd notch to create the mild contraction required.

If you are practicing your Pilates exercises at home, take a few simple steps to ensure a trouble-free session.

- Turn off the phone
- Choose a time when you will not be interrupted
- Have anything you need close at hand – water, etc.
- Move all furniture away from the immediate area
- Make sure you have a mat or towel to cushion the spine
- Ensure the space you are using has sufficient ventilation and the temperature is appropriate.

Pelvic floor

Another option to engage the deep abdominal muscles is to activate your pelvic floor. Recent research has proved that the transversus abdominis and pelvic floor co-activate. When you initiate one the other is also activated. So you have a choice. It is important that you don't engage both together as this will create too strong a contraction in the deep abdominals and reduce the stabilising effect of these local muscles, usually resulting in too much global activity.

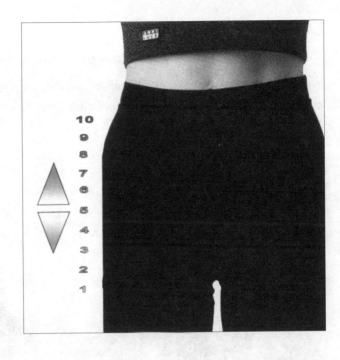

- To engage the pelvic floor muscles, imagine you desperately need the bathroom and there isn't one available.

- Think about a lift going to the 10th floor – breathe out and tighten your pelvic muscles a little at a time at each floor until you reach the 10th floor. Breathe in and release completely.

- Now breathe out and tighten your pelvic muscles a little at a time to the 10th floor again and release to the 5th floor..

- Next breathe out, bring the lift to the 10th floor, release to the 5th and then to the 3rd floor to the base level of engagement. Release completely.

- Finally, draw the lift directly to the 3rd floor and try to maintain this engagement throughout the exercises.

It doesn't matter which method you use – either transversus abdominis drawing in to the 3rd notch of an imaginary belt, or, through the pelvic floor, drawing the imaginary lift up to the 3rd floor – what is important is that you remember you only engage one or the other, not both together.

LATERAL BREATH

The final piece of this stability jigsaw is the part played by the lateral breathing technique.

In order to keep the neutral spinal alignment and mild engagement of the deep abdominals, a lateral breathing pattern is the best way to allow free flowing, functional movement to occur.

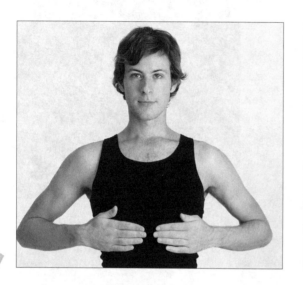
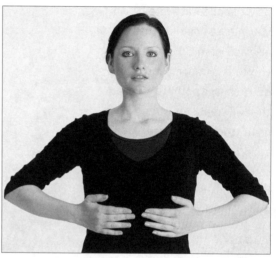

To work with a lateral breath you will need to pay attention to your ribcage, how it expands and contracts as you breathe in and out.

- Place your hands on the front of your ribs with the fingertips touching.

- Inhale, feel your ribs expand and notice if your shoulders rise up as you inhale. If this does happen, try to stop it occurring and focus on the expansion of your ribs.

- As you exhale, notice how the ribs close down and narrow.

- As you breathe in and out, ensure that your belly does not push out.

Good shoulder posture

Now that you are on the road to establishing pelvic stability, you need to consider the upper body, which is also important to the golf swing and to spinal health.

Think about the position of your shoulder blades. Notice if you carry a lot of tension around the neck and shoulders. In order to stabilise your shoulder girdle to reduce the potential for injury whilst playing golf, you will need to become aware of your shoulder blade alignment.

Stand tall and allow your shoulder blades to melt down your back. Notice how this allows the chest to rise and open and that your neck automatically lengthens.

This openness in the chest and increased volume helps to create a stable shoulder girdle that in turn will alleviate any old shoulder injuries and reduce the risk of further problems

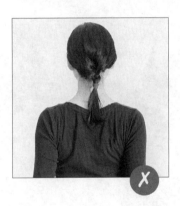 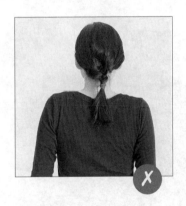 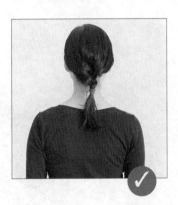

With your neutral spine, mild engagement of the deep abdominals, lateral breath and shoulder stability you are now all set to begin your Pilates Institute Method programme.

It's a good idea not to rush this initial process. Before you begin the programme, do your best to understand this set up and sequencing.

One of the easiest ways to practice this set up is to do so whilst you are just walking around doing everyday things.

This will help you to become familiar with the "feeling" of being in your best alignment.

Practice the stance when you get ready for your set up to take a swing, Notice how it changes your address to the ball and maybe increases the acceleration of the ball.

Whether you are an amateur or a professional, take care to notice the effect these changes have on your game. It could be almost immediate. If you are taking professional tuition, it is advisable to speak to your golf professional and let him or her know that you are working on your postural stability.

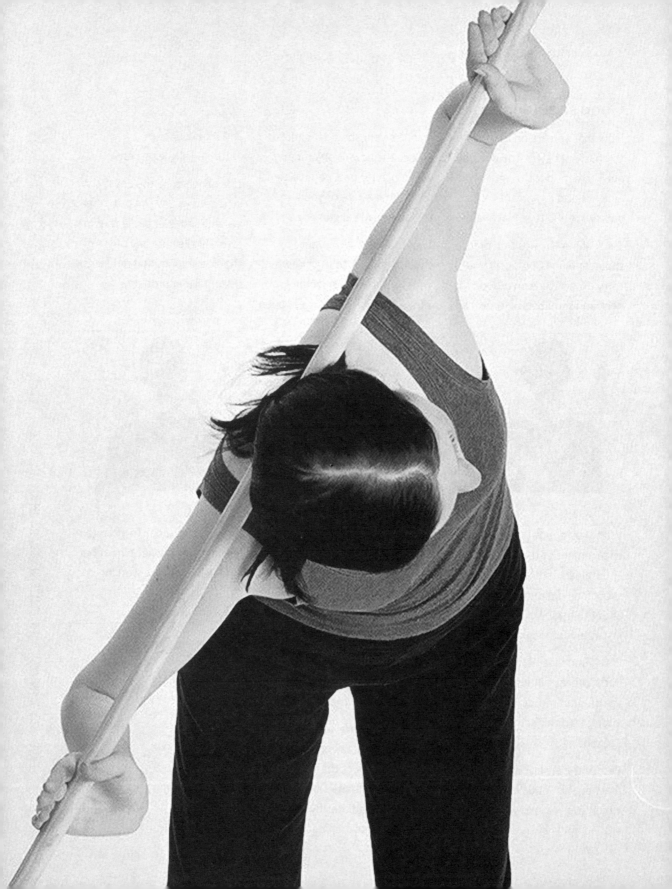

pre-game preparation

PRE-GAME PREPARATION

Warming up in preparation for your game of golf is important not only to improve your game but also to help prevent injury.

It is a common misconception that golfers don't need to do anything other than play the game. Among the processes some neglect in addition to general fitness is an effective warm up.

A survey of over 1,000 randomly selected amateur golfers from different golf clubs in Melbourne, Australia in June 1999 confirmed that most golfers don't warm up.

More than 70% of the sample said they never or seldom warmed up, with only 3% stating they warmed up on every occasion they played. (*Journal of Science and Medicine in Sport 6.*)

The most common reasons given for warming up were:

- Improved play (74.5%)
- Injury prevention (27%)
- Because everyone else did

Common reasons given for not warming up were:

- No need (38.7%)
- Lack of time (36.4%)
- Can't be bothered (33.7%)

Warming up before playing is important, especially as there is a growing number of older players enjoying golf in their retirement.

Of course professionals have a higher rate of injury, but amateurs are usually less well conditioned and therefore place greater stress on their bodies from the repetitious nature of the game.

So warming up is important for everyone playing at all levels. An effective warm up for golf would include some aerobic activity to raise body temperature, stretching for your "golf" muscles and joints – wrists, hands, arms, shoulders, lower back, chest, trunk, hamstring and groin – and finally using a progressive golf swing to gradually increase range of motion in the trunk.

PRE-GAME WARM UP EXERCISES

Set up stance

We recommend you begin your preparation time by spending a few minutes finding your neutral spinal alignment, mildly engaging your deep postural muscles and confirming a lateral breathing pattern.

This set up stance will enable you to stabilise your pelvis and shoulder girdle ready for the round.

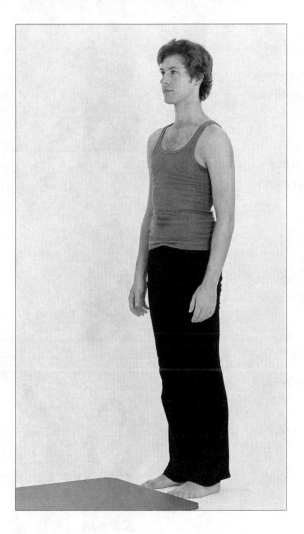

- Stand tall with your feet hip width apart

- Rock your pelvis backward and forward and slowly come to a position where your pelvis sits between the two extremes of tilt.

- Engage your inner unit by either drawing in your navel to the third notch on your imaginary 10-notch belt, or drawing the imaginary lift up to the third floor of the 10-storey building. Only engage these postural muscles with one connection to ensure the engagement is mild and constant.

- Allow your shoulders to ease away from your ears, thinking about creating a soft V shape between your shoulder blades. It might help to think of the shoulder blades as two ice creams melting down your back.

- Once you have achieved your set up stance, do your best to maintain this connection and alignment throughout your preparation. Stabilising your pelvis and shoulder girdle will allow for safe and effective movement patterns to develop.

- By focusing on your alignment, postural support and breath, you will connect with the mindfulness of your game from the start.

ARM CIRCLES

- Stand in your set up stance.

- Connect your inner unit by gently contracting your deep abdominal muscles.

- Slowly start to rotate your shoulders – up to your ears, backward and down then forward. Don't force the rotation, just allow the shoulders to release.

- Gradually allow the arms to get involved with the movement, starting with circling the elbows and then lengthening the arms.

- Breathe evenly as you release your shoulders blades down your back and float your arms out in front of your body. Gradually bring the arm up to your ears and rotate the shoulders to bring the arms around and return to the start.

- Continue these full arm circles for 10 repetitions, breathing in as you start the circle and out as you open the arms and complete the circle. Start with a backward motion and then reverse.

- Take care not to create unnecessary tension in the shoulders or neck.

- Coordinate the movement with the breath and allow the length of your breath to determine the speed of the movement.

Why?

- Warms up and lubricates the shoulder joint by increasing blood supply to the shoulder area

- Prepares the shoulders for a full range of movement in the swing action

- Gives the golfer an improved chance of having an easy full swing at the start of play

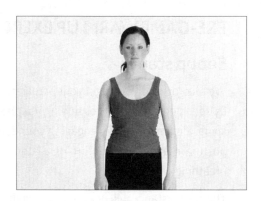
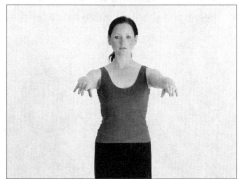
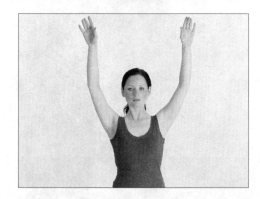
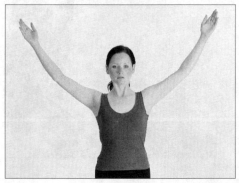

OVERHEAD RAISE

- Stand with your feet shoulder width apart with your neutral alignment and postural muscles working.

- Hold a club with your hands just a little wider that your shoulders.

- Melt your shoulders down your back as you raise the club overhead. Make sure your shoulders stay away from your ears by stabilising your shoulder girdle and creating the soft V between the shoulder blades.

- Bring the club back to the start position and repeat the overhead raise.

- Repeat the movement for 10 repetitions.

- Breathe in as you raise the club and breathe out as you lower it.

- Focus on the inner unit staying connected and the shoulders melting down.

Why?

- Prepares the shoulders for a better top-of-backswing position

- Improves range of motion in finish position or follow through

- Increases leverage on the downswing from the top

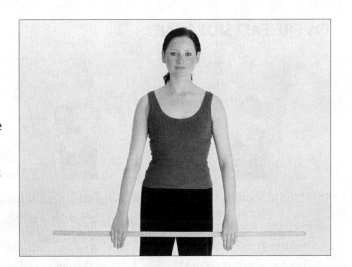

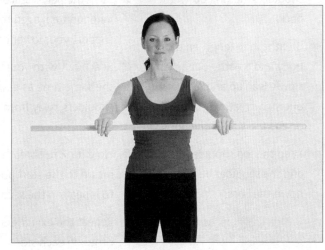

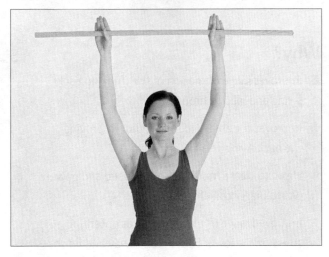

OVERHEAD SIDE BEND

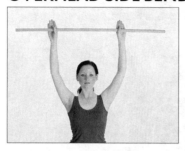 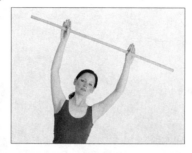 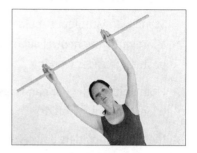

- Stand in your set up stance.

- Hold the club as for the overhead raise with shoulders melting down the back.

- Breathe in to lengthen the body and breathe out as you slowly lean up and over to one side, creating a stretch on the top side of the body.

- Keep the top shoulder back and the shoulder blades down the back.

- Keep your neck equally long on both sides – try not to rotate the head.

- Keep the pelvis still and inner unit engaged to support your lower back.

- Reach out with your arms at the same time as easing the shoulders away from the ears

- Hold for 2 full breaths and return to the start position to repeat on the second side.

- Repeat the exercise 3 or 4 times on each side.

- Take care with this movement. Move into position with focus and notice any discomfort in your lower back.

- If this position aggravates existing lower back or shoulder issues, modify it by not holding the club overhead but placing one hand on your hip for support and slowly raising the top arm overhead to create the stretch. Only stretch as far as your can control the position, (see 2 pictures below).

Why?

- Improves range of motion of the trunk on back swing and follow through

- Improves the ability to rotate, thus improving the back swing

- Helps to create more club head speed and power with a bigger coil effect

- Improved range of motion reduces potential stress on the lower back in take away and finish

SUPPORTED SIDE BENDS

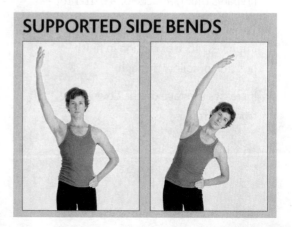

ROTATIONS

(only to be performed if you don't have any lower back or shoulder issues)

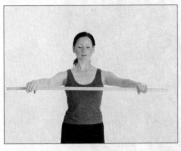 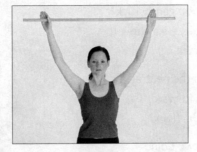 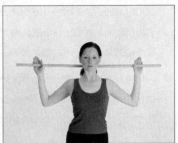

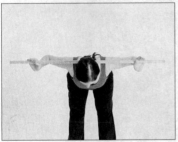 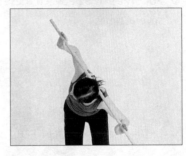

- Holding the club at each end, slowly melt the shoulders down the back and raise the club behind your head. If this position is not possible due to shoulder or neck issues, place your arms in a "surrender" position with arms at a 90 degree angle.

- Bend from the hips – no lower than 90 degrees. Ensure that your pelvis is in a neutral alignment and your inner unit is supporting your lower back.

- Rotate the upper body from side to side.

- Keep the lower body stabilised and still.

- Repeat the exercise 10 times each side.

- Stop if you feel pain or discomfort in the lower back.

Why?

- Prepares golf-specific muscles for any aggressive movements, especially at the start of play

- Prepares the body for the correct sequencing of the swing whilst warming the muscles

- Improves the ability to stabilise during the swing from the start, creating better quality of play early in the game

HIP MOBILISERS

- Standing with legs hip width apart, soften your knees and breathe out as you gently tuck your pelvis under (a backward tilt). Be aware of the lengthening in your lower back.

- Allow the pelvis to drop back to the neutral position and then tilt the pelvis forward, tipping the hip bones towards the floor.

- Rock the pelvis between these two points several times.

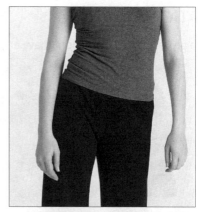

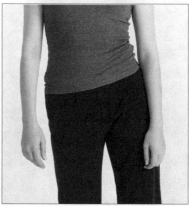

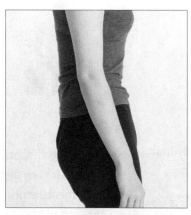

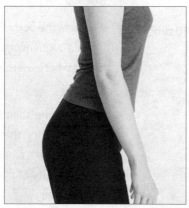

- Now imagine a string hitching your hips up towards the ceiling.

- Swing them from right to left.

- Now incorporate all the moves together – tilting backward, then to the side then forward and finally to the second side.

- Keep the knees soft and rotate the pelvis several times to the right and then repeat to the left.

Why?

- Improves mobility in the lower back, decreasing the risk of lower back injury

- Improves mobility in the hip area to avoid degenerative arthritis of the hip

ROLL DOWNS

- Stand in your set up stance.

- Hold the club at either end in front of your body.

- Breathe in to lengthen the spine and breathe out as you bring your head to your chest and start to roll down through your spine.

- Allow the club to hang away from the body.

- Bend your knees when you feel tension in the lower back or hamstrings.

- Ensure your postural muscles are engaged to support the lower back.

- Lead with the head and let the neck feel long.

- At the bottom of the movement, slowly re-stack the spine vertebra by vertebra from the bottom, melting the shoulders away from the ears until you return to the standing position.

- Don't force this movement. Allow the weight of the body to help with the stretch.

Why?

- Improves forward mobility of the full spine, reducing the risk of injury

- Creates a more relaxed posture

- Having a better range of movement in the spine will improve your swing

- Improves the depth of your breathing

- Roll downs can be used to gauge the flexibility of your spine ready for your pre-game warm up

- Improves shoulder stability

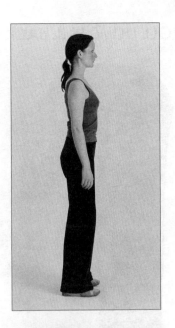

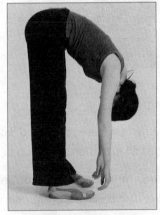

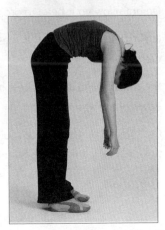

49

ROLL DOWNS & BACK EXTENSIONS

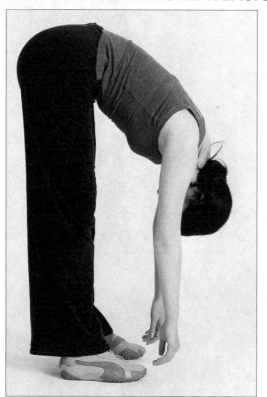
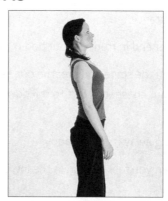
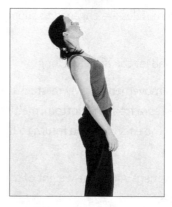
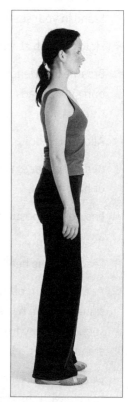

- When you have completed 3 or 4 roll downs (forward flexion) then add an extension at the top of the movement.

- Breathe in and imagine you are lifting your ribs off your waist and bending backward over a pole underneath your shoulder blades,

- Do not allow your head to drop back uncontrolled.

- Feel the stretch across the chest and the long muscles in the back working.

- Breathe out and lift the chest back onto the ribs to start your roll down phase again.

- Complete 3 or 4 complete movements rolling down (forward flexion) and leaning back (extension).

Why?

- Mobilising the back helps withstand the excessive torque from early swings

- Creates a more relaxed posture

- Increases the mobility of the spine decreases the risk of injury to the lower back early in the round

- Stretching around the back of the hips maintains flexibility to avoid pain and injury

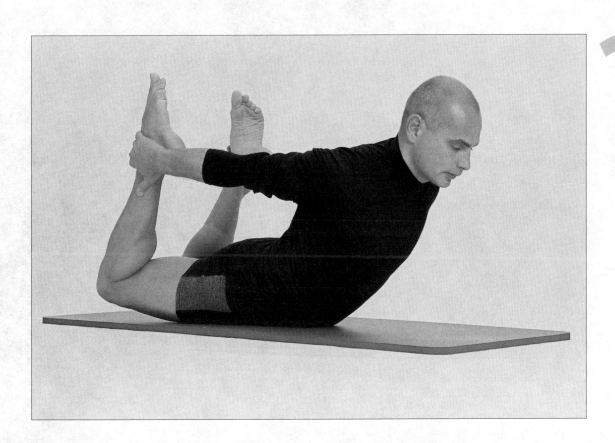

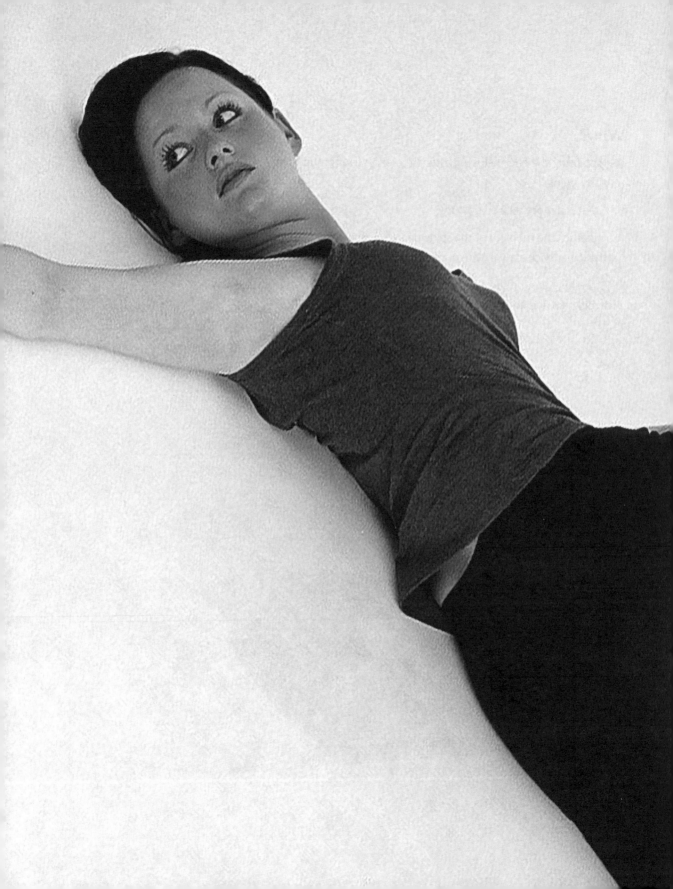

Squats

- Stand with feet shoulder width apart in your set up stance.

- Hold the club at each end in front of the body.

- Lower the body by using a sitting position.

- As you sit back into the squat position, allow the arms to float forward to counterbalance the weight.

- Keep the upper body long and stabilise the shoulder blades by melting them down your back.

- Keep your head in line with your spine – don't flex your neck.

- Repeat this exercise up to 10 times.

- Ensure your heels stay on the floor even if this limits your range of motion.

- Keep your inner unit connected to support your lower back.

- Breathe out to start the squat, breathe in at the bottom of the movement and use the power of the out breath to drive your legs and buttocks to bring you back to a standing position with the arms coming back to the start position.

- Should you feel any pain or discomfort in your lower back, check your posture and if necessary reduce the number of repetitions.

Why?

- Good overall warm up for muscles

- Improves the range of motion in the hips

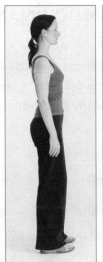
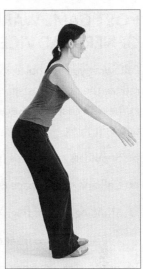
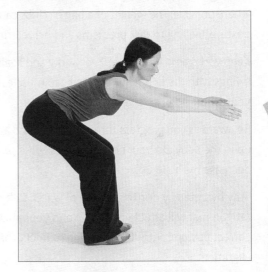
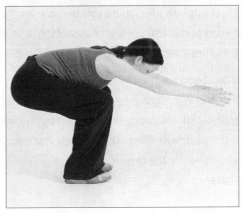

53

POST GAME WARM DOWN AND GENERAL ADVICE

Following your 18 holes, it is important to warm down to help reduce the risk of post-game stiffness or soreness. Use the stretches in the next chapter, particularly those listed below, immediately upon finishing.

- Shoulders and triceps (page 62)

- Calf and soleus (page 65)

- Standing back of thigh (page 65)

- Kneeling hip and front of thigh (page 67)

Try not to carry your bag around the course, but push it in a trolley where possible. The weight of a bag of clubs can seriously affect your posture, leading to disk problems and nerve irritation.

Keep your game functional. Every now and again try a few practice swings with the opposite hand to keep muscles balanced and keep your whole body involved.

Be aware as you progress through your round about tension building up in the body. Do your best to address your posture or stance to decrease the build up.

Stay hydrated by drinking plenty of water. Dehydration causes fatigue that will affect your game and your ability to hold your correct posture, potentially leading to injury through poor alignment.

Most importantly, should you become aware of pain or discomfort that is persistent, see a specialist. Attend to your health before it becomes a serious problem.

Whilst you are healthy and enjoying your game, the Pilates Institute Method will play a large part in keeping you strong, flexible and mobile. Should you need to attend to injuries at any time, the Pilates Institute Method will teach you how to get back in the game and maintain the rehabilitation carried out by your physical therapist.

"We should recognise the mental functions of the mind and the physical limitations of the body so that complete coordination between them may be achieved."

(Joseph Pilates)

stretching for golf   55

STRETCH FOR GOLF

The balance between mobility and stability for a golfer is key.

Having too much of either can result in a lack of control or power. Adequate stability is needed to direct the force of the swing with control whilst working within the normal range of joint mobility and muscular flexibility.

Stretching offers a profusion of choices. How should we stretch? For how long? How long will it take to develop the stretch? How long will the effects last?

There are many theories and heaps of research into this element of fitness. For our purposes we want to look at the major muscles involved in the game of golf and guide you with some no-nonsense stretches that will help you to develop and maintain a normal range of movement through your joints and muscles.

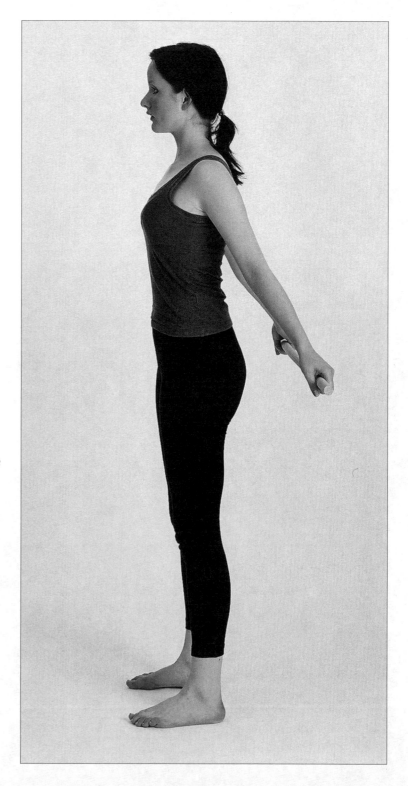

Golfing Muscles

- Front of thigh (quadriceps)
- Back of thigh (hamstrings)
- Outer thigh (abductors)
- Buttocks (gluteals)
- Waist (internal and external obliques)
- Lower back (erectors)
- Mid/upper back (latissimus dorsi, rhomboids, trapezius)
- Chest (pectorals)
- Shoulder (deltoids)
- Rotator cuff (infraspinatus, teres minor, subscapularis, supraspinatus)
- Back of arm (triceps)
- Front of arm (biceps)
- Forearm (forearm flexors and extensors)

All the major muscles are used during a round of golf. These muscles need to be strong to enable the body not only to effectively play the game but also to have a balance of mobility and flexibility to avoid overuse injuries and give the maximum results.

So which stretch should you perform on a regular basis in order to develop your flexibility, and what do you need to do to maintain the improvements?

Muscles respond best when they are warm and pliable. Before your round of golf it would be wise to stretch the muscles gently following some exercise to raise the temperature of your body – a brisk walk to the course would suffice. Once your round is complete, some muscles may feel tense and shortened and will need lengthening before their temperature cools and cause stiffness.

Basically there are two type of stretching:

Maintenance Stretching

This type of stretching is held for just 6–10 seconds. Take the muscle to the point of tension, hold for the required amount of time and release. Muscles that require this type of mild stretching are those that do not need to be lengthened for optimal function.

These muscles, assuming they are healthy and have no injuries requiring special attention are:

- Neck
- Shoulder
- Front of arm
- Back of arm
- Abdomen
- Front of thigh
- Buttocks
- Shin
- Soleus (lies underneath the belly of the calf)

Developmental Stretching

This type of stretching is held for a longer period of time: 15–30 seconds. If you stretch for more than 30 seconds at one time, ligaments may become compromised. If you feel that you want to focus on extended stretching, then release the stretch position every 30 seconds to take the strain from the ligaments that are stabilising the joints.

Take the muscles to the point of tension, just the same as with maintenance stretching. Hold the point of tension until the sensation of stretch wears off, then take the stretch further until the sense of tension is felt again.

Never force a stretch, but always work within the limits of your flexibility. If shaking occurs, release the position immediately back to a point of no shaking. Whilst being stretched, muscles should remain relaxed and you should breathe deeply.

Muscles that benefit from developmental stretching are those that are used in such a way that they shorten during daily activities. If you drive a lot or sit for long periods at the computer, muscles at the back of the legs, at your hip joints and chest will shorten and tighten and if ignored may create postural problems, headaches or lower back pain.

Muscles that may benefit from developmental stretching are:

- Chest
- Muscles either side of the spinal column
- Hip flexors
- Back of thigh
- Inside thigh
- Calf (belly of the muscle)

Both maintenance and developmental stretches are termed "static". Do not bounce into the stretch as this will have the opposite effect that you need. Bouncing into a stretch confuses the reflex that allows a muscle to release and lengthen and so this only results in mis-communication between the brain and the muscle, the consequence of which is shorter muscles for most people.

Remember that with all developmental stretches, it is not advised to hold the stretch for longer than 30 seconds at any one time. By all means repeat the stretch following a 10 second break, but be aware that you do not want to overextend the ligaments that are needed to hold the joints in a stable position.

the stretches

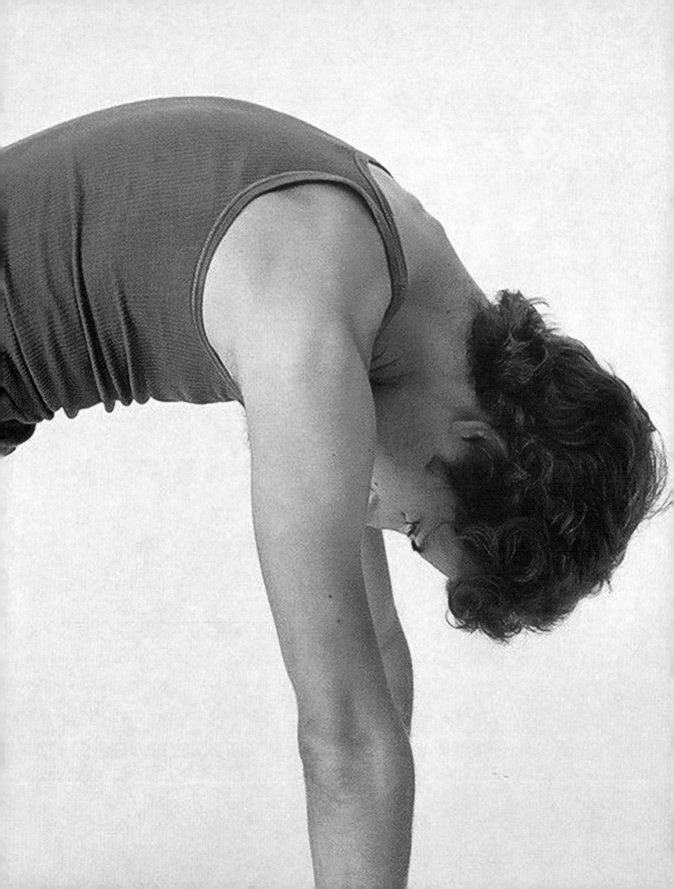

Maintenance Stretches

NECK STRETCH

Standing or sitting with good posture, allow your right ear to ease towards your right shoulder feeling a mild stretch along the side of the neck. Breathe in and allow the left shoulder to gently lengthen away from the left ear. Hold this stretch for 5–10 seconds and return your head to the upright position. Repeat on the left.

NECK ROTATION

Standing or sitting with upright posture and inner unit connection, ease your shoulder blades down your back – without causing undue tension in the neck – and slowly turn your head to the right. Only turn to the point of tension and then return to the start position to repeat on the other side. Repeat this 3 times each side.

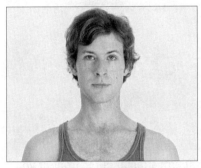

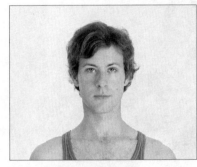

Why?

These stretches will help improve your posture and reduce the risk of neck injury with your swing

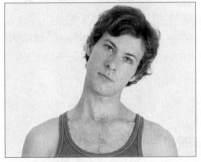

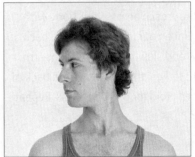

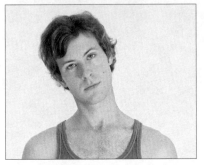

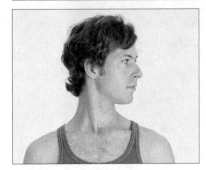

SHOULDER AND TRICEPS

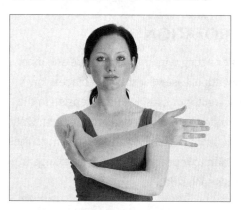

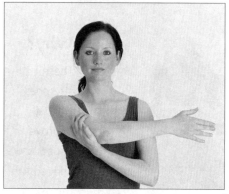

Standing or sitting, reach across your body with your right arm. Place your left hand on the back of your right elbow and slowly ease your right arm towards your chest. Feel the stretch at the back of the right shoulder. Hold for 6–10 seconds. Repeat for left shoulder.

Why?

Helps with shoulder flexibility and assists your back swing and follow through

WRIST FLEXORS

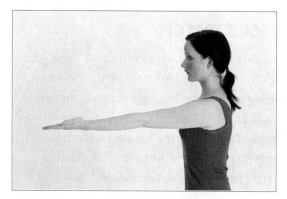

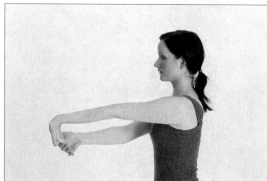

Extend your right arm straight out in front of you with the palm up. Hold onto the fingers with the left hand and gently bend the wrist down. Feel the stretch in your forearm. Hold for 6–10 seconds. Repeat for the left arm.

Why?

Helps prevent golfers elbow

MAINTENANCE STRETCHES

TRUNK ROTATION

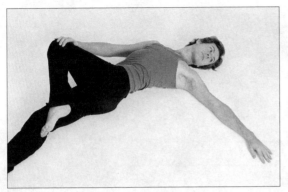

Lie on your back with both legs straight. Bend your right knee and take it over the straight left leg. Keep your shoulders on the floor. Breathe in, and as you breathe out gently press the left leg towards the floor. Feel the stretch in your lower back and chest as you turn your head in the opposite direction and keep your shoulders on the floor. Hold for 6–10 seconds. Repeat on the other side.

Why?

Helps increase rotational range in your lower back, assisting your swing and reducing the risk of injury.

FRONT THIGH

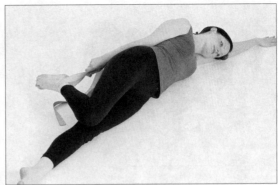

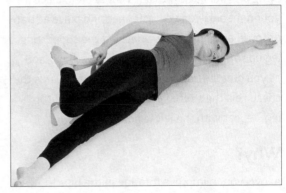

Lying on your side, wrap a towel or strap around your top ankle. Bend your top leg at the knee to 90 degrees. Gently bring your pelvis into a backward tilt by easing the tailbone under and imagine the top knee is lengthening away from the hip joint. At the same time, slowly draw the heel of the top leg towards the buttocks. Hold for 6–10 seconds. Repeat on the other side.

You can also perform this stretch standing so that you balance on one leg or use a chair or wall for support.

Why?

Counterbalances the effects of a forward tilt of the pelvis, reducing the risk of low back pain.

BUTTOCKS

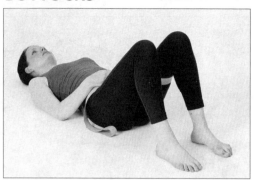

Lying on your back with both knees bent, place your right ankle on your left knee and place a strap or towel around the under leg. Lift the supporting leg up so the knee is over the hip. Breathe in, and as you breathe out press the under leg towards the chest. Feel the stretch in the buttock of the top leg. Repeat with the left leg on top.

Why?

Allows you to improve rotation in the hips to improve your swing

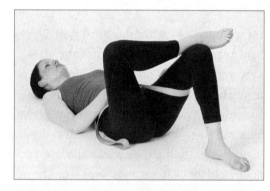

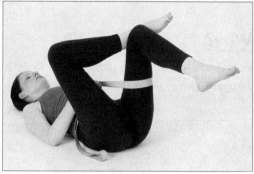

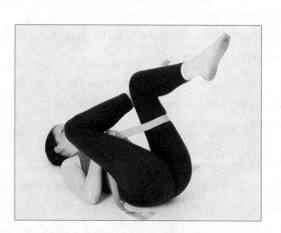

CALF

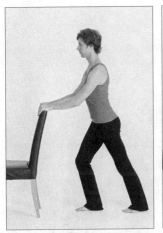 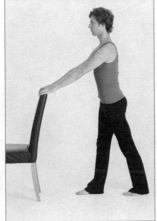

Stand facing a chair or wall for support. Take your right foot behind you by stepping back onto the heel. Lean forward slightly, feeling the stretch in the fleshy part of the calf muscle.

Hold this stretch for up to 30 seconds. Change legs.

The calf muscle benefits from Developmental stretching.

SOLEUS

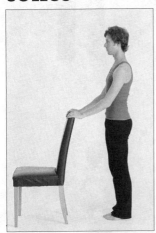 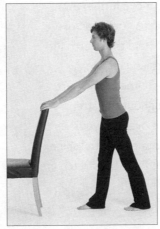

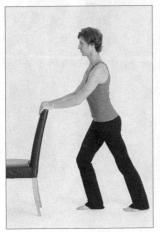 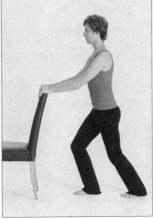

The soleus muscles lies underneath the main calf muscle and can only be stretched if the knee is bent.

Begin by re-visiting the calf stretch set up. You may need to bring your back foot closer to enable you to bend the knee and keep the heel on the floor.

Stand facing a chair or wall for support. Take your right foot behind you by stepping back onto the heel, feeling the stretch in the fleshy part of the calf. Slightly bend the knee of the stretched leg, keeping the heel on the floor. Feel the tension move down to the heel. Imagine your heel reaching out behind you.

Hold this stretch for 6–10 seconds. Change legs. It is recommended that you practice these two stretches in combination to ensure addressing the complete calf area.

Why?

To reduce the risk of injury (Achilles Tendonitis).

Developmental stretches

CHEST

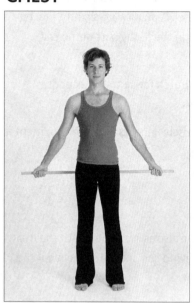

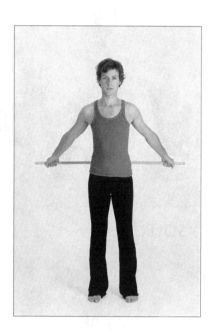

Stand with your golf club behind your back at hip height with your hands facing forward. Check your set up. Breathe in and reach your hands away from the hips. As the hands move further away, you will feel a stretch across the chest. Hold the stretch for 30 seconds and release. Repeat 2–3 times. Make sure that throughout this stretch you do not overarch your back. Maintain a neutral spine and do not force the stretch or hold your breath.

Why?

Helps with a general improvement in posture and help prevent shoulder injuries.

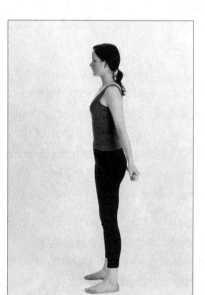

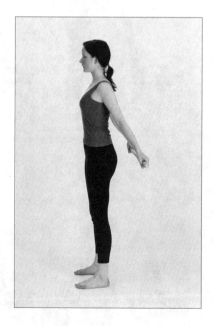

Muscles of the Back

CAT STRETCH

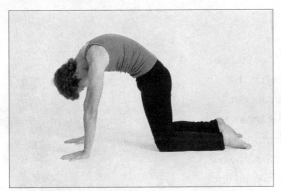

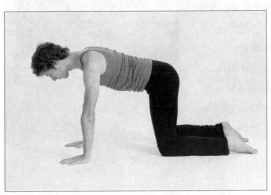

Kneel on all fours, with legs apart, ensuring wrists are under shoulders and knees are under hips. Set up your neutral spine and stabilise your shoulder girdle. Breathe out and tuck your tailbone under as you drop your head and arch your back. Feel the stretch in the upper and lower back. Breathe in and return to the neutral start position. Repeat this 4–5 times.

Why?

Helps avoid injury and improve your swing

HIP AND THIGH STRETCH

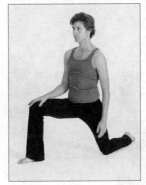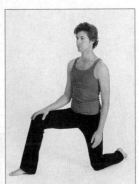

Kneel down and place your right foot flat on the floor in front of the hip. Ensure the knee is directly over the heel. Tilt your pelvis under and gently lean back until you feel a stretch in the front of the hip joint. You may also feel the stretch down the front of the thigh. Hold for 30 seconds and release. Change legs.

Repeat on both legs 2 or 3 times.

Why?

Improves your posture and reduces the forward pull on your pelvis, thus reducing the risk of low back pain

Back of Thigh

STANDING

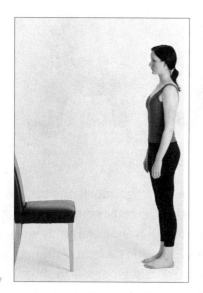

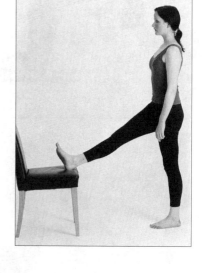

Using a chair, bench or golf cart, place your right heel on the seat. Make sure you are not forcing down on the knee cap. Take a deep breath in and feel the spine lengthen. Breathe out as you lean gently forward until you feel a stretch at the top of the back of the leg. Hold this stretch until the sensation of tension wears off (about 30 seconds) and then ease a little further into the stretch until the feeling of tension re-appears. Change legs. Repeat on both legs once more.

It is OK to bend the knee if the stretch feels extreme, especially if you are only feeling it in the calf or behind the knee.

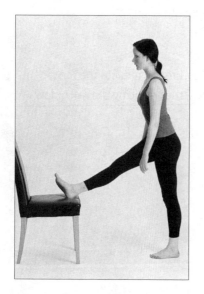

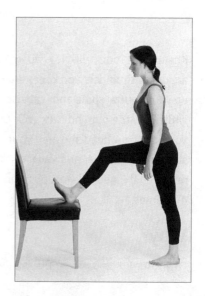

LYING ON THE FLOOR

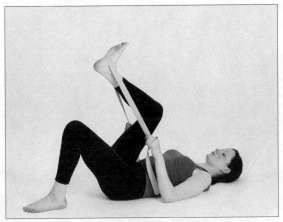

If you are very inflexible you may prefer to stretch your hamstrings lying down, using a towel or strap. Lie with both knees bent. Place a strap/towel around your right foot and lift the leg up, keeping the knee bent. Slowly begin to lengthen the leg until you feel a stretch at the back of the thigh. Bend your knee if the leg shakes or you only feel the stretch in the calf or back of the knee. Hold this stretch for 30 seconds and then release for about 10 seconds and repeat the stretch sequence. Change legs. Repeat on both legs one more time.

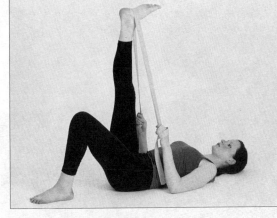

Why?

Improving flexibility in the hamstrings allows you to maintain your neutral posture and reduces the strain on the lower back during your game of golf

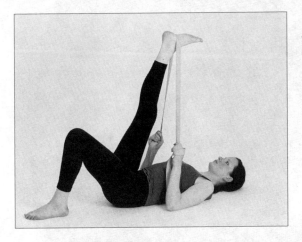

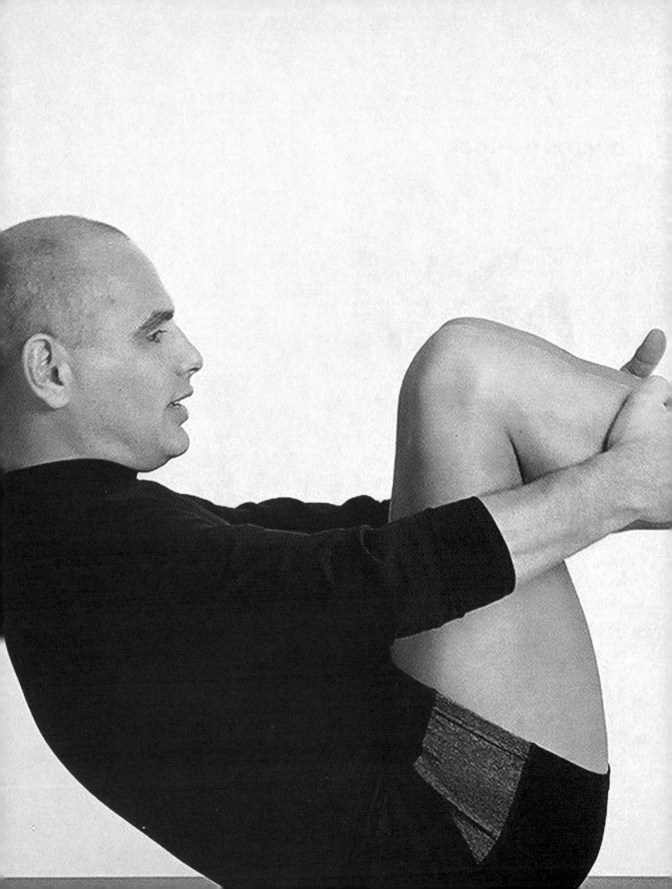

the movements

PUSH UP

This movement challenges the flexibility of your spine together with the strength of your back muscles, shoulder girdle and core.

- Stand in the set up position with feet hip width apart

- Find your neutral pelvic alignment and engage your deep abdominal muscles

- Soften your knees

- Breathe in to grow tall then slowly bring your chin to your chest to start the rolling down element of this move.

- Gradually curl your body towards the floor, your head leading the way

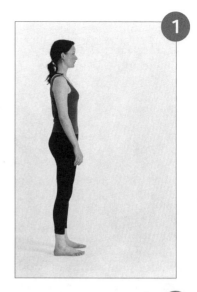

- Use the support of your hands on your thighs if you experience a sense of stiffness in your lower back or the back of your legs.

- Breathe out, bend your knees, place your hands on the ground and walk them out until you are in a box position

- Your hands are under your shoulders

- Your knees are apart under your hips

- CHECK YOUR SET UP – do you still have a neutral spinal alignment? Are your shoulders easing away from your ears? Is the mild connection to the deep abdominals still engaged?

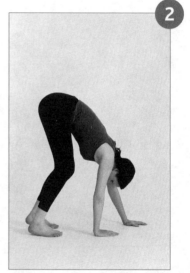

Why?	Strength and flexibility
How?	One continuous movement
Watch Out!	
Bend your knees	
Don't force this movement	
Check your shoulders stay down	
Reps	5–10 times
Visual	Wallpaper peeling off a wall

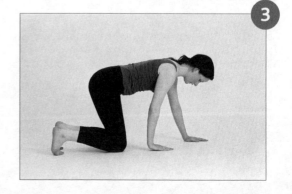

- Breathe in as you bend your elbows to lower your body towards the floor

- Only go as low as you can maintain good alignment with your shoulders remaining wide and flat

- Breathe out to straighten your arms

- Walk your hands back toward your feet

- Bend your knees to ensure your heels return to the floor before you begin to uncurl your spine – vertebra by vertebra – until you have returned to standing

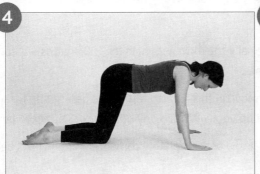

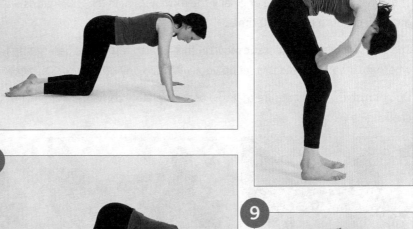

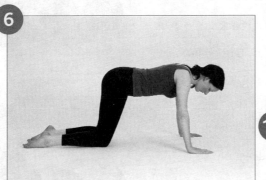

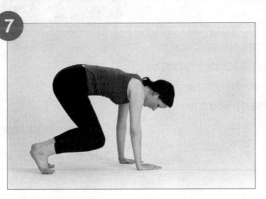

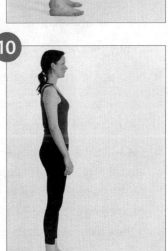

73

THE HUNDRED

The 100 is so called because originally the move was held for 100 breaths – breathing in for 5 counts and out for 5 counts a total of 10 times.

The 100 set up is the only static move in this repertoire. It is the base set up for several movements and when you have mastered this set up you will find many other moves easier to perfect.

Do not rush the levels; ensure that you are completely competent at one level before attempting a more challenging version.

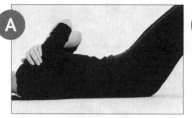 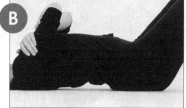 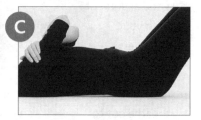

- Lie with your knees bent

- Lengthen your neck (gently bring your chin towards your chest without raising your head off the ground)

- Melt your shoulders down your back

- Allow this action to release any tension in your upper back and chest

- Find your neutral spine

- Gently press your lower back into the floor

- Now arch it in the opposite direction

- Allow it to settle at the mid-point between these two extremes

- You will sense a space between your back and the floor. It may not be a real space as this will depend on the shape of your spine. However, there should be a feeling of lightness as though you could place a grape there without squashing it.

- Engage your inner unit (core)

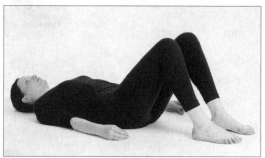

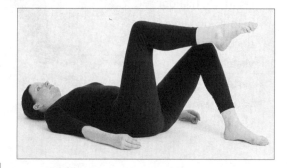

- Focus on lateral breathing (see p. 38)

- Keep your spine long and breathe naturally

- THIS IS THE BASE SET UP FOR THE 100

To challenge yourself in this position you may now attempt to lift your right leg to a 90 degree angle with the knee directly over the hip.

- Ensure that the weight of the leg does not affect your neutral set up

- Your deep abdominals should stay connected

- Your superficial abdominals (those close to the surface) should not push out (dome)

- Hold this position for 5 complete breaths in and out

- Now allow the leg to unfold towards the floor

- Revisit your set up and repeat on the left leg.

When you can hold this position steadily for 20 continuous breaths you may want to increase the challenge.

- Gradually begin to straighten the lifted leg until you feel an increase in the weight, challenging your ability to maintain the set up.

- Decrease the breaths to 10 or 15, gradually working your way back to 20 breathes

The next level of challenge will be to raise both legs.

- Lying supine in the set up position, float the first leg to a 90 degree angle

- Gently allow your lower back to press into the mat for safety

- Lift your second leg

- Return to a neutral spine

- Hold the position for up to 20 breaths

- Allow your breathe to remain natural

When you have completed your challenge, allow your lower back to rest on the floor and lower the

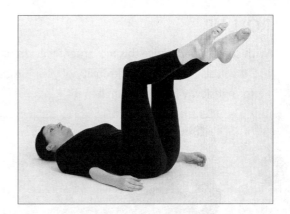

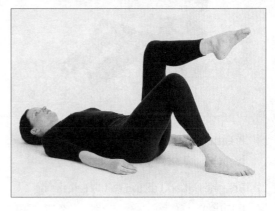

legs one at a time. Return to the set up position.

Why?	Strength and stability
How?	With control

Watch Out!

Ensure your hips stay level as you lift and lower your leg

Keep your leg at a 90 degree angle

Don't allow your lower back to press into the floor

Reps	5–10 times
Visual	Raised leg like a table top

ROLL UP

With consistent practice this movement will strengthen core muscles and superficial abdominal muscles too. It will also improve the flexibility of your lumbar spine. This movement requires control and focus. Perform it slowly for maximum benefit.

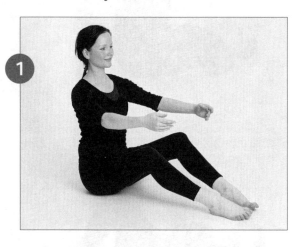

- Start in a seated position at the end of your mat
- Sit as tall as you can
- You may need to sit on a rolled up towel if your back muscles are stiff

- Breathe in, start to tilt your pelvis under and begin to roll slowly backwards
- Breathe out and return to the tall sitting position
- Gradually make the movement bigger, creating a bigger challenge
- Only go back as far as you can control this movement

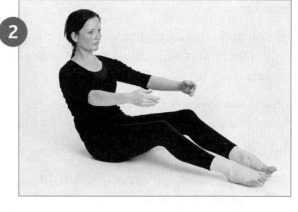

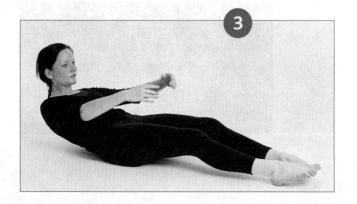

- If you start shaking, or your feet lift off the floor reduce the size of the movement
- You can use 4 breaths
- If the movement become too large to be completed in two breaths.

ROLL UP PROGRESSION

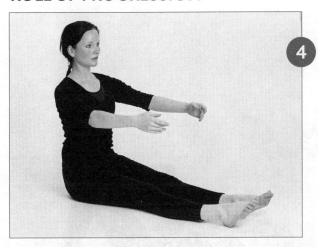

4

- Breathing in to grow tall
- Breathing out to pelvic tilt and lengthen towards the floor
- Breathing in at the bottom of the movement
- Breathing out to return to the tall sitting position

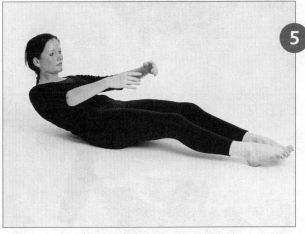

5

Why?	Core strength and flexibility in the lumbar spine
How?	Start with a pelvic tilt and slowly lower yourself down

Watch Out!

Keep your shoulders down

Don't poke your chin forward

Reps	5–10 times
Visual	Lowering yourself slowly into a hot bath

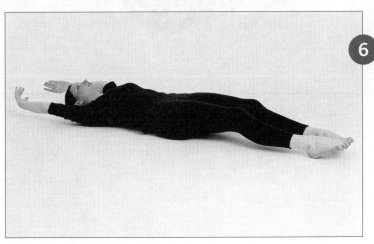

6

ONE LEG CIRCLE

This movement will eventually improve hip mobility. The set up is the same as the first level position for the 100.

- Raise your leg to a 90 degree angle – knee over the hip joint

- Ensure you have your set up in place – neutral spine and mild connection of the deep abdominals

- Start to make small circles in the hip joint towards the centre of the body

- Imagine you are drawing circles on the ceiling with a pencil attached to your knee

- Focus on the control required to maintain the set up as the hip rotates

- Breathe in at the start of the circle and out as the leg moves further away

- When you have completed 5 rotations in one direction, reverse the movement

- Check the leg that is not circling does not rock or roll.

- Try to make the circles equal in size

- Repeat on the other leg.

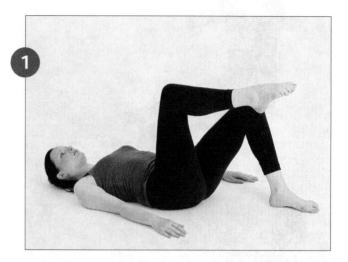

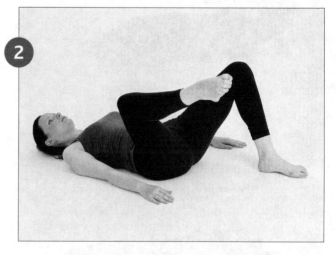

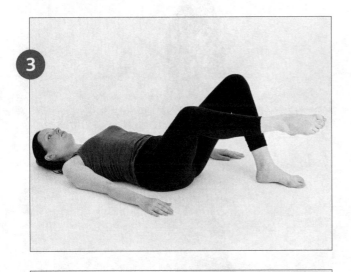

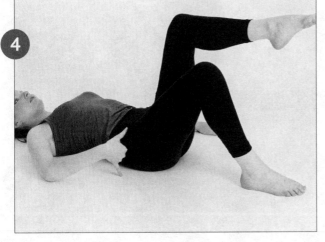

Why?	Mobility in the hip joint
How?	Making sure the hips don't move

Watch Out!

Keep the raised leg at 90 degrees

Maintain a neutral spine

Reps	5 circles in each direction
Visual	A pencil on your knee drawing circles on the ceiling

ROLLING LIKE A BALL

This movement will mobilise the spine and strengthen your core. Because it uses the weight of the body to create the rolling movement, you will need to focus on controlling the speed with shoulder and pelvic stability to avoid unnecessary momentum.

If you know your lower back is stiff, use your arms to assist the performance.

- Sit tall at the end of the mat

- If you need to, place your hands slightly behind your hips

- Otherwise place them softly on your shins but don't grip

- Connect your core muscles

- Breathe in and start to roll back by tilting your pelvis under

- Roll back as far as your shoulder blades only – NOT ONTO YOUR NECK

- Immediately roll back to seated

- Repeat 5–10 times

- As you gain confidence you can start and finish the movement in a balanced position with your feet hovering off the mat and your hands on your shins.

- Try to imprint each section of your spine onto the mat as you roll back and forth

- To increase this challenge, slow the movement down and use control and focus

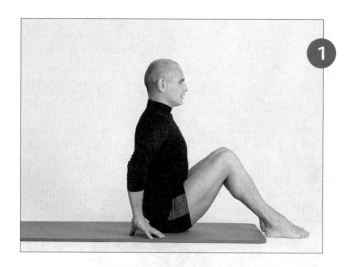

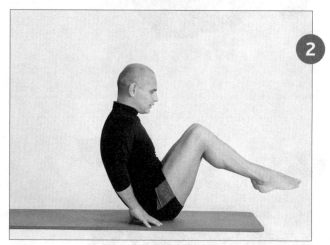

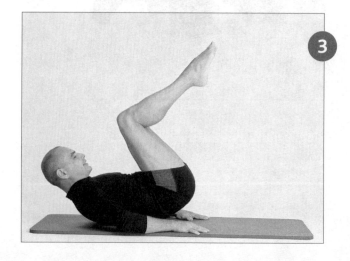

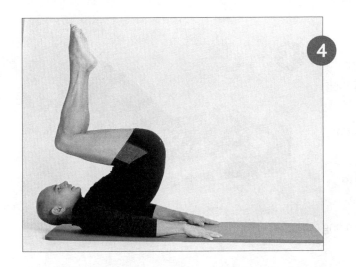

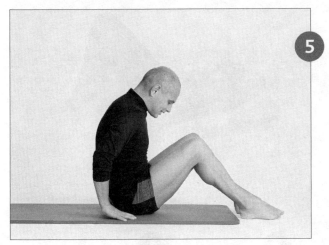

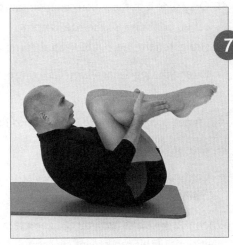

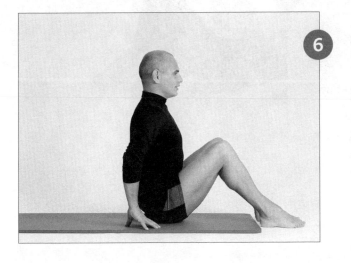

Why?	Mobility of the spine
How?	With control from the base of the spine to the shoulder blades

Watch Out!

Don't roll onto your neck

Reps	5-10 times
Visual	Rocking chair leg

SINGLE LEG STRETCH

This movement will challenge your ability to maintain the set up position whilst moving your legs. It will help to strengthen your core.

- The set up for this move is the base position of the 100

- Place your fingertips on your hip bones to check for unnecessary rocking of the hips

- Breathe out and start to slide your foot along the ground away from the body

- Only slide it as far as you can maintain the set up position – so the goal is not to straighten the leg, but to keep alignment.

- Extend the leg as far as you can control the set up position

- Immediately return it to the start position.

- Repeat with the other leg

- Continue alternating the legs whilst maintaining stability in the hips.

When you are confident you can complete 10 repetitions of this movement successfully, you may want to increase the challenge.

The next level of this movement starts in the same position as level 1 of the 100.

- Lie with your knee over your hip in the set up position with a neutral spine

- Slowly start to extend your toe towards an imaginary door bell

- The lengthened leg will appear heavier, requiring more control

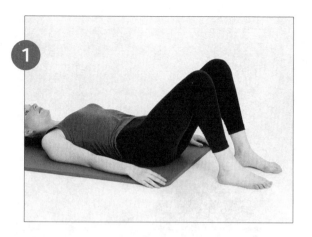

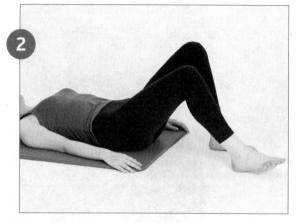

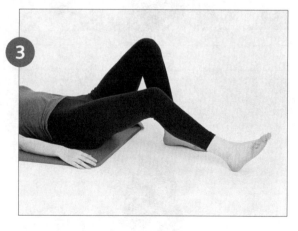

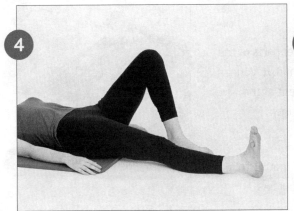

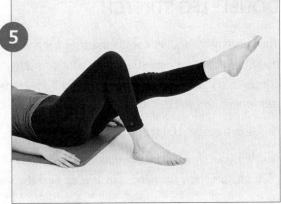

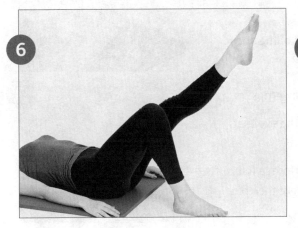

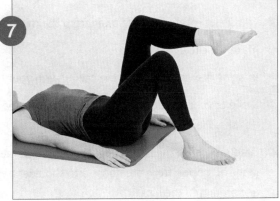

- You don't have to straighten the leg, just increase the length to a point where you feel a greater challenge

- A 45 degree angle will create a greater challenge.

- Perform repetitions on each leg

- Take care when changing legs that you maintain the set up

Why?	Core stability
How?	With control

Watch Out!

Keep hips even

Ensure you keep neutral alignment

Reps	5–10, alternating the legs
Visual	Sliding your heel through wet sand

DOUBLE LEG STRETCH.

This movement requires control in the upper and lower parts of the body. Eventually you will strengthen your core and improve your coordination. We will start with the upper body element of the movement. This will help to mobilise your shoulder joints.

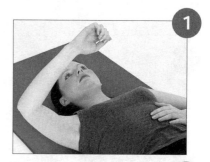

- Lie in the base 100 set up position

- Melt your shoulders down your back and allow your arms to float up so that the hands are directly over the shoulders

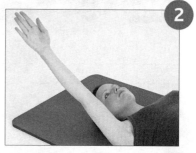

- In this position begin to make small circular movements with your arms

- The circles rotate outward away from the mid line of the body

- Make the circles equal in size

- Imagine drawing circles on the ceiling with your fingertips

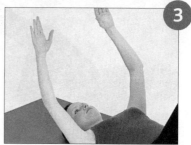

- If one of your shoulders is stiff, make both circles the size that this shoulder can cope with.

- Gradually make the circles larger until you can perform a full range of motion from the floor up to shoulder height then out and around to the hips

- Only make the circles as large as you can without your ribs rising up

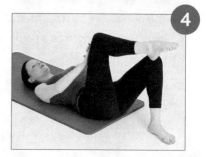

- You should not feel a stretch in your back

- Don't worry if you can't make a full range circle, but work to your available mobility in the shoulder joint

- Breathe in at the start of the circle and breathe out as your arms move away from the body

- Complete 5–10 circles

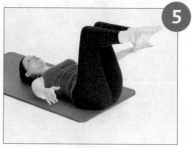

When you can complete 10 circles with control of the upper body and ribs together with maintaining the neutral setup in the spine, you may want to add a strength challenge – by using the arms only we have been mainly mobilising the shoulder joints although we have been engaging our core muscles too.

To add a significant strength challenge:

- The set up position is the same as the base of the 100

- With your right leg at 90 degrees and maintaining the set up, start to circle the arms whilst the leg stays still

- Perform 5–10 circles and change legs, taking care to keep the set up

- Repeat using the other leg as the strength challenge.

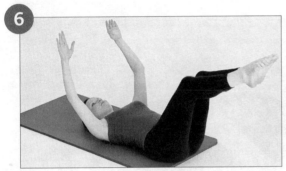

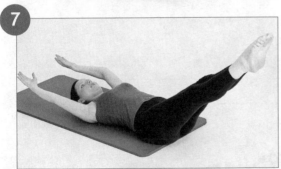

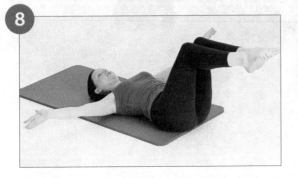

When you can control the upper and lower body equally and are able to make a full circle with the arms, you can add the challenge of coordination to this movement.

Do not rush these levels – make sure you can keep your ribs down as the arms go behind the head for the full range of movement.

- Starting position is the same as the level 1 100

- As you start to circle the arms up and back, begin to extend the right leg that is at 90 degrees to about a 45 degree angle

- Breathe out as the arms and leg move away from the body

- Breathe in as the arms and leg return to the start position

- Ensure the leg comes back to 90 degrees with the knee over the hip

- It is important that you coordinate the movements of the arms and leg, which should open at the same pace and return to the start position at the same time

- Use the breath to assist the speed and control of the movement.

- Repeat using the other leg

Why?	Core strength and shoulder mobility
How?	With control
Watch Out!	
Keep ribs soft	
Don't lose neutral set up	
Reps	5–10 times
Visual	An elastic band being pulled in opposite directions

SWAN DIVE

A common postural issue is rounded shoulders because we sit for long periods of time using computers and driving. This movement will help to mobilise the mid-back whilst strengthening the muscles we need to maintain good posture.

This movement is in prone (lying on your front). If this causes discomfort in the lower back, place a rolled up towel underneath your hips – it may help.

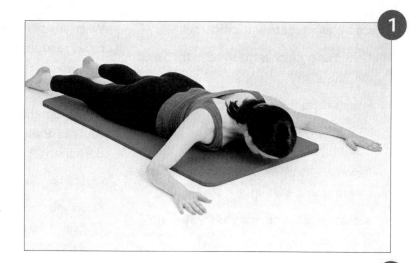

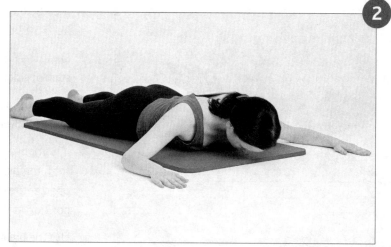

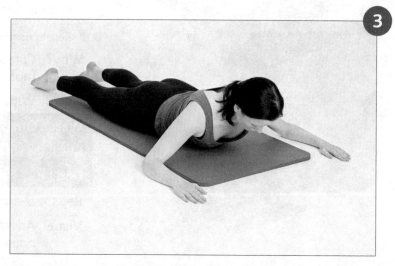

- Lie on your front with your arms in the "surrender" position

- Your legs will be hip width apart

- Relax your buttock muscles

- Tilt your pubic bone gently toward the mat and find your neutral spine

- Engage your deep abdominal muscles – imagine a flame underneath your navel as you draw it away from the mat

- Slide your shoulder blades down your back

- Lengthen your neck and imagine you are a tortoise coming out of its shell

- Breathe out as you slowly start to peel your breastbone, head and shoulders off the mat

- Breathe in as you melt your ribs back down onto the mat

- Ensure that you don't push on your arms to force you up higher than you can naturally move

- Avoid tension in the lumbar spine

- Focus on lengthening rather than lifting

- Keep your gaze on the floor at all time and don't flex your neck

- Repeat this movement 5–10 times

It may take you several repetitions to decide what is the correct level for you – take this time as it is important you do not over-extend your lower back.

IF YOU HAVE ANY SPINAL DISC ISSUES, OSTEOPOROSIS OR ARTHRITIS, CHECK WITH YOUR MEDICAL PRACTITIONER WHETHER EXTENSION TYPE MOVEMENTS ARE SUITABLE FOR YOU

Why?	Mid-back mobility
How?	Focusing on lengthening the spine

Watch Out!

Don't push hip bones into the floor

Keep shoulders down

Don't push on forearms

Reps	5–10
Visual	Like an aeroplane off the runway

SIDE KICK

This is a balance challenge – for some, just lying on their side will be sufficiently challenging whilst they attempt to maintain the neutral spine, mild engagement of the deep abdominals and lateral breathing.

If you find that the set up for this position is enough at the moment then stick with it and master the challenge of side lying before you move on to the various balance challenges.

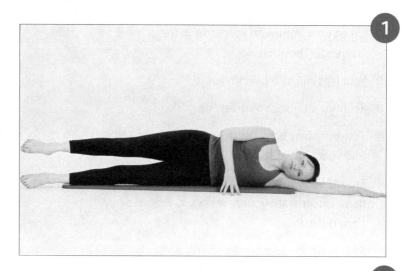

- Lie on your right side with your head resting on your lower arm and the fingertips of the upper arm gently resting on the floor in front of the chest

- If you need to, place a cushion between your ear and your upper arm. This will help to keep your neck in a good position without strain

- Stack your shoulder, hips, knees and ankles

- Ensure you can see the tops of your feet

- Your body set up should be the same as in standing

- When you are aligned, engage your core muscles

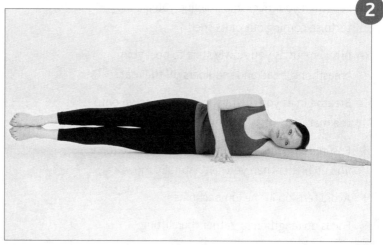

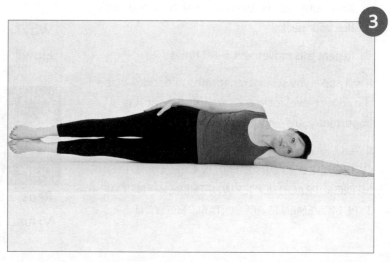

- Lengthen in both direction, reaching out from your centre to your toes and from your centre to the tips of the fingers of your lower arm

- Draw your waist away from the mat – imagine you are lying on a sheet of ice

- If you can maintain this position without wobbling, start to move the fingertips of the top arm closer to the body – this will create a bigger balance challenge

- If you can maintain this position, place your top arm on to your thigh

- Maintaining this position, start to lengthen the top leg until it floats away from the bottom leg – keep this leg still. IT IS IMPORTANT THAT THE WAIST STAYS CONNECTED. DO NOT HITCH THE HIP UP – WORK FOR LENGTH

- Maintain this position for 5–10 breathes

- Repeat on the other side

If this position is challenging you sufficiently and you really have to concentrate to maintain your balance, stay with this level until it is easily achieved. When you can hold this position for the required time, you are ready for an additional strength and balance challenge.

- Lie on your side with your top arm on your thigh and the top leg floating away from the bottom leg, head resting on your lower arm

- Breathe out and lengthen the lower leg

- It may float up to meet the top leg – this will increase the strength and balance challenge

- Now you have to support the weight of both legs in a balance position

- Make sure this does not make you wobble or cause you low back discomfort. If it does then return the lower leg to the floor

- Maintain this position for 5–10 breaths

- Repeat on the other side.

Make sure that you take time with setting up this movement. When you change sides you may find the two sides of your body do not respond identically – allow for this difference by taking your time to achieve optimum set up position.

Why?	Balance and core strength
How?	In sequence
Watch Out!	
Make sure you can see your feet	
Don't put too much pressure on the stabilising hand	
Don't hold your breath	
Reps	5-10 times
Visual	Lying on the edge of a wall

SCISSORS

This movement will strengthen the deep abdominal muscles. Move with control and progress gradually.

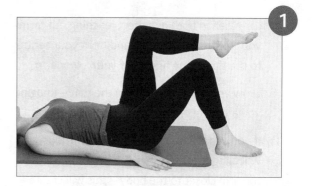

- Lie on your back in the base 100 position

- Breathe out to float up your right leg up to a 90 degree angle

- Concentrate on maintaining your neutral set up

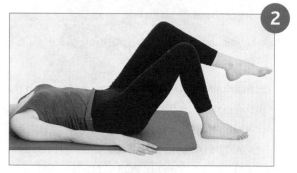

- Breathe out and start to move your foot towards the floor

- Keep the shape of the leg constant

- Only move your leg as low as you can keep the neutral set up

- When you have reached the lowest point that you can control or tapped the floor, breathe in to immediately return the leg to the 90 degree position.

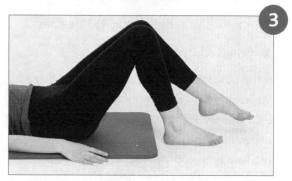

- Repeat this hinging movement 5–10 times, breathing out as the leg moves away and breathing in to return the leg to the start position.

- Repeat on the other leg

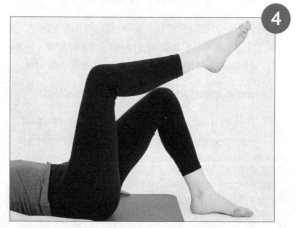

SCISSORS PROGRESSION

When you can successfully repeat this movement 10 times on each leg, you are ready for the next level of challenge.

- Using the same set up and action, start to gradually open out the angle of the knee, creating an increased challenge with the weight of the leg

- Repeat on the second leg

When this effort become less challenging, you can consider trying the next level.

- Lie on your back in the base position for the 100

- Breathe out and float the right leg up to 90 degrees with the knee over the hip

- Breathe in to pause a moment and breathe out to return the leg to the floor

- Breathe in to change to the other leg and repeat the action

- Continue to alternate the legs – making the changeover when both feet are on the floor

The challenge is in the changeover; ensure the hips do not rock.

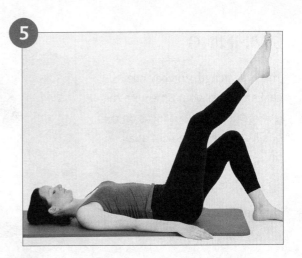

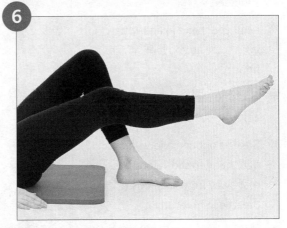

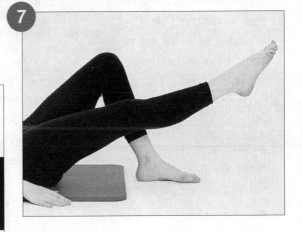

Why?	Core strength and toning for the legs
How?	With coordination

Watch Out!

Keep the angle of the leg constant

Don't lose neutral alignment

Reps	5–10 times
Visual	Dipping your toe into water

SWIMMING

This is a strength and balance challenge. Take your time with the levels. Don't rush, but focus on the quality of the movement at all times.

- Kneel on your mat on all fours

- The knees are under the hips

- The wrists are under the shoulders

- Keep your head in line with your spine as you look at the floor

- Find your neutral spine and engage your core muscles

- Breathe out and allow your right hand to slide along the mat away from the body. Breathe in to return

- If you can maintain alignment without hunching the shoulders, allow the arm to float up – no higher than shoulder height

- When you have achieve a good level of movement quality alternating right and left arms, repeat the action with your right leg

- Breathe out imagine your big toe pushing through wet sand as your right leg slides along the ground. Breathe in to return

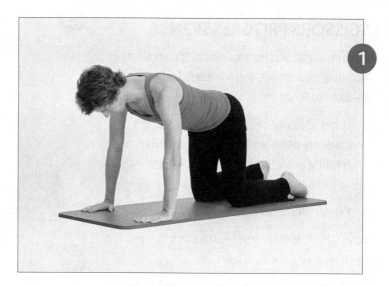

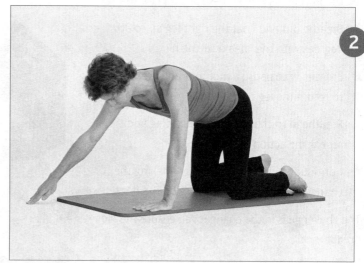

- Alternate the legs, making sure you maintain the set up of the torso.

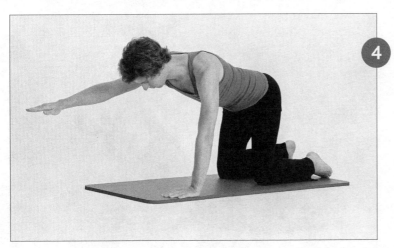

When you can slide the legs and arms separately, you are ready to combine the two movements.

4

- Maintain the all fours position, focusing on good alignment

- Breathe out to allow the right arm and left leg to slide simultaneously away from the centre, breathe in to return

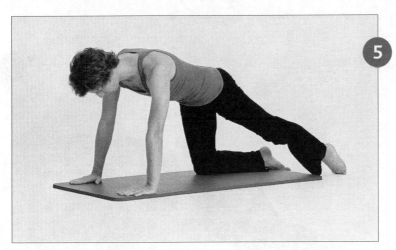

5

- If you can maintain good quality of movement, allow the arm and leg to float away from the body, increasing the balance and strength challenge

- Alternate sides 5–10 times

Why?	Strength and balance
How?	In opposition from the core

Watch Out!

Don't lean from side to side

Keep head in line with spine

Keep shoulders away from ears

Reps	10, alternating legs
Visual	Tray of glasses on your back

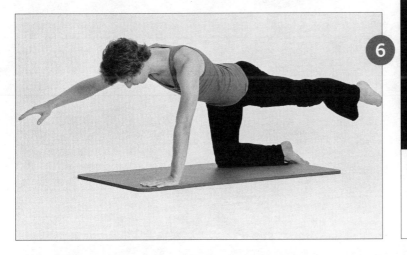

6

SIDE BEND

This is a challenging set up position. Ensure the set up is correct before attempting the movement element.

- Lie on your side with your elbow under your shoulders, knees bent at 45 degrees

- Check that your heels, hips and elbows are in line

- Engage your deep abdominal muscles

- Make sure both sides of your waist are equally long

- Don't allow the underside of the waist to sag – imagine a helium balloon supporting it at all times

- Keep the shoulders melting down your back and the chest wide

- The fingertips of your top hand should hover just above the floor

- Breathe out and try to lift your hips straight up to the ceiling

- Think about a hoist connected to your top hip pulling you straight up

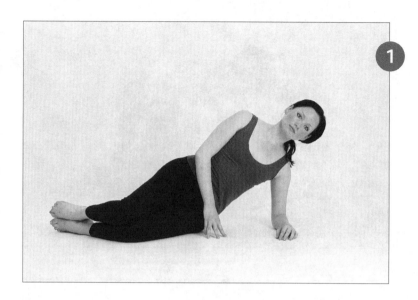

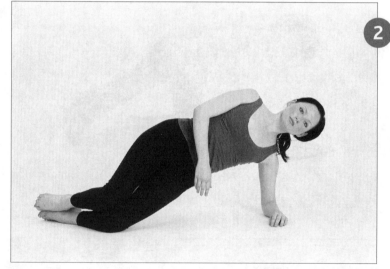

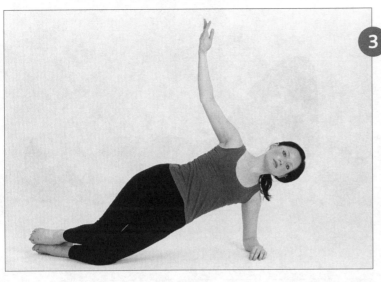

3

- Breathe in as you gradually return to the floor

- Don't relax. Just touch the floor very lightly before repeating the movement

- Keep your neck long at all times and in line with the spine

Build the repetitions gradually, always making sure that the alignment is excellent. This will alleviate any problems with the shoulders and neck.

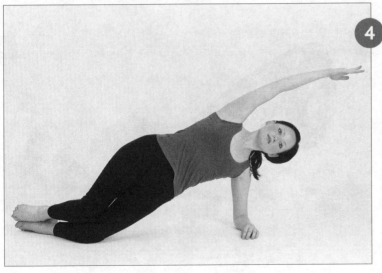

4

Why?	Strengthen shoulder girdle and stretch waist
How?	Keeping heels, hips and elbow in line

Watch Out!

Just lightly touch the mat as the hips come down

Keep shoulders wide and flat

Don't lean into support hand

Reps	5–10 times
Visual	A hoist from the ceiling

SHOULDERS BRIDGE

This is a perfect movement for those with stiff lower backs. Do not place anything under your head when performing this movement to avoid placing pressure on your cervical spine.

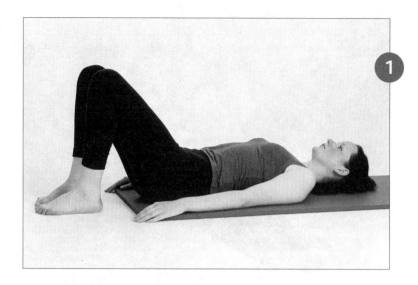

- Lie on your back in the base set up for the 100

- Start with a neutral spine

- Breathe in and allow your lower back to tilt backwards to the floor

- Breathe out and return to neutral alignment

- Tilt your pelvis backwards and begin to lift your hips off the mat towards the ceiling

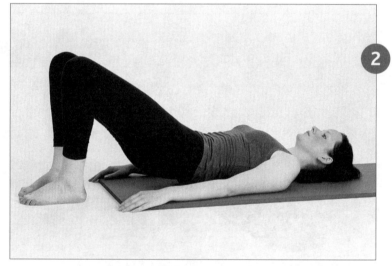

- The highest you will lift your hips is the ski slope position – when the knees, hips and shoulders are in line

- Don't lift so high that you feel tension in your low back or push your hips forward

- Return to neutral spine each time you lower to the mat

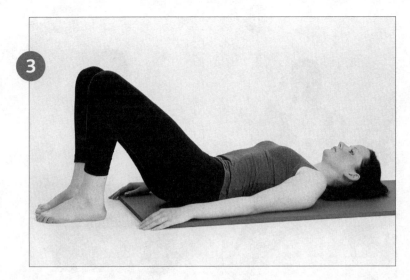

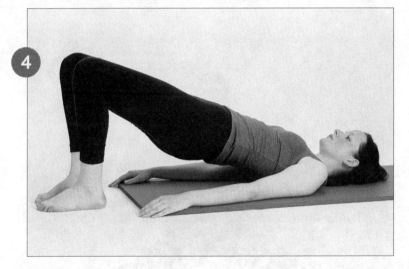

As the movement gets bigger you will need to use a 4 breath count.

- Breathe in to wait
- Breathe out to pelvic tilt and peel the spine up to the ski slope
- Breathe in at the top
- Breathe out to melt the spine back down to the neutral position

Sometime it just feels good to practice the beginning of this movement, pelvic tilting and returning to neutral. For those with stiff lower backs, it's a great release.

97

Why?	Lower back mobility
How?	Disc by disc
Watch Out!	
Keep knees in line	
Don't press on the neck	
Reps	5–10 reps.
Visual	Like a chain link

SPINE TWIST

This movement is great for golfers. It challenges the core with rotation and extension, both of which are used extensively in golf. It is also very beneficial for older adults as the ability to rotate well is something that diminishes as we grow older.

● Sit on the floor or in a chair with the legs hip width apart

● Sit as tall as you can

You have three choices for the arm positions:

1 Sitting with the thumbs against the breastbone will help keep the shoulders in good alignment

2 Sitting with the arms in a "Cossack" position is more challenging but will still allow the neck and shoulders to bear less weight

3 Sitting with the arms fully extended to the sides is the most challenging

You have also three choices for the leg positions:

1 Sitting with the soles of the feet together

2 Sitting with the knees bent

3 Sitting with the legs straight out in front

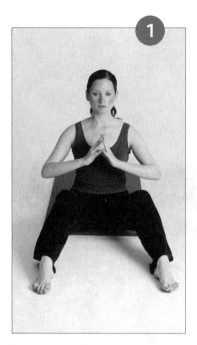
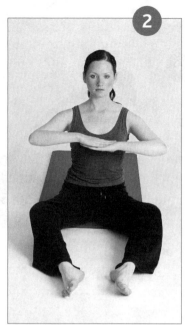
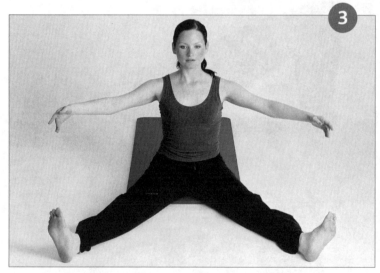

Decide on the arm and leg position that you will be able to maintain throughout the movement.

● Sit tall and ensure that both buttocks stay firmly on the floor, breathe out as you start to slowly rotate to the right

● When you reach a point of tension

● Breathe in and return to the start position

4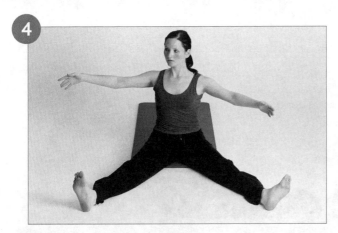

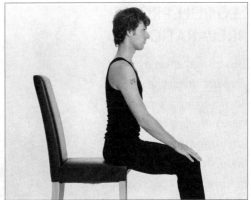

5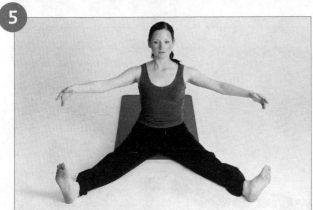

- Repeat on the other side

- Alternate sides 5–10 times

- Don't allow the arms to swing past the point of rotation

- Keep the head in line with the spine at all times and move the torso as one piece

- Don't allow the head to move independently of the body

- Focus on not only rotating but also lengthening through the spine with each repetition

6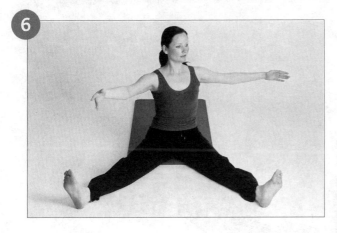

Why?	Mid-back mobility
How?	Rotating and extending the spine

Watch Out!

Keep both buttocks on the mat

Move the spine as a whole

Soften knees

Reps	10, alternating sides
Visual	Like a corkscrew

LEG PULL PRONE PREPARATION

This movement is a preparation for the more advanced leg pull prone and is known in yoga as the plank. It is a total strength move. Should you have any shoulder or lower back issues, you may prefer to work with the set up position only.

- Lie in a prone position (on your front)

- Assume a sphinx position with your elbows directly under your shoulders

- Tilt your pubic bone towards the mat

- Come into your neutral spine position

- Engage the core muscles

- Melt the shoulder blades down your back and stabilise the upper body

- Hold this position for 10 breaths

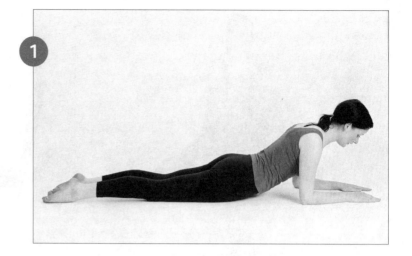

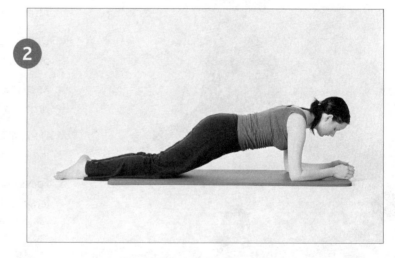

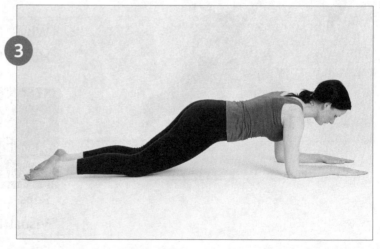

When you can successfully hold this position without undue stress on the shoulders and neck or lumbar spine, you can attempt the next level of challenge.

- Lengthen from the centre out through the legs and up through the upper body

- Lift the hips off the floor

- In this lifted position, make sure your core muscles are supporting your lower back

- Hold the position all the time you can maintain good alignment

There should be not unnecessary straining with this movement.

Why?	Strength
How?	With precision
Watch Out!	
Don't let hips sway forward	
Keep shoulders away from ears	
Lengthen neck	
Reps	Hold the position for 30–60 seconds
Visual	Like a plank

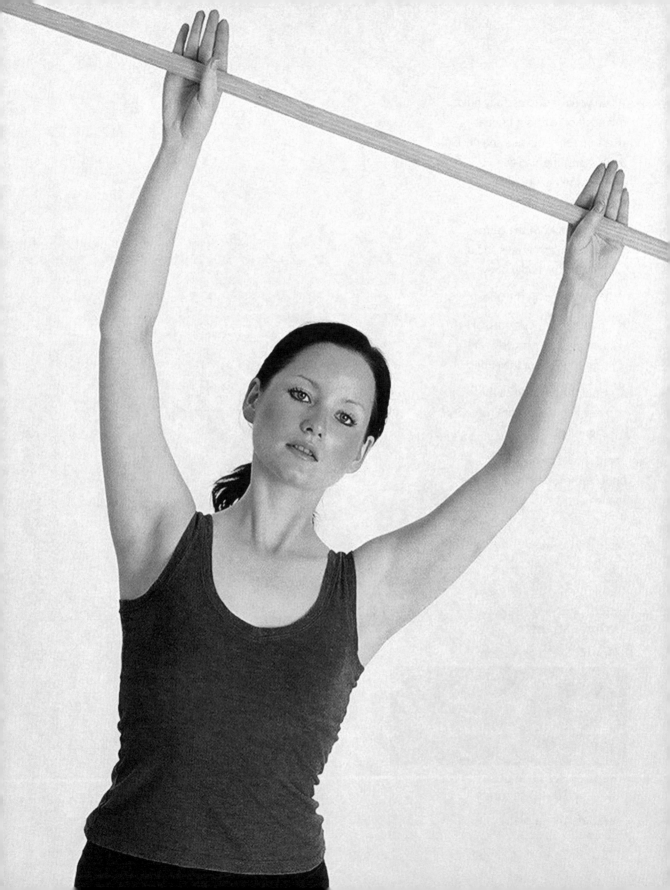

the programmes

The programmes

The programmes offered are not based on your current fitness levels but on your experience, practice and understanding of the Pilates Institute Method.

Take your time, not only to enjoy your practice, but to fully understand how your body is responding to the movements. Only when you are able to carry out the exercises with precision and control, should you think about moving to the more challenging levels.

Your main aim is to improve your game of golf – so take time when you are playing to notice how your body responds to the various positions you need to place yourself in.

Strength and flexibility in combination with appropriate mobility and stability are the important areas.

Use your practice to improve your awareness and understanding of your body.

ALL EXERCISES ARE NOT THE SAME

Don't worry if some of the movements are more difficult than others. Every body is different and each day can see changes depending on the activities you have undertaken. You will find some exercises easier in the evening, as you have been active all day and so the body is more mobile. Take each day as it comes and do the best you can at each practice session.

DON'T RUSH

The programmes have been divided into Levels 1, 2 and 3. These are just a guide. Eventually you will want to design your own programmes. Just make sure when you start to develop your own programmes that they are a balance of strength and mobility exercises and that your body is not over worked in one area. Keep to the principles of Pilates, and be true to the technique's philosophy of mind, body and spirit.

NO TIME?

If time is a problem, choose the exercises that you find most beneficial and spend 10 or 20 minutes of practice. Don't forget you can apply the Pilates Institute set up of neutral spine, gentle connection and lateral breathing to everyday activities such as walking, sitting and standing in line. Of course, when you have time you can enjoy a full, dedicated Pilates practice session.

THE LEVELS

From the start of your practice try to remember the names of the exercises. This will help you create smooth transitions to each exercise.

You don't have to launch immediately into a prescribed session. You may find it useful to take each exercise and practice individually before trying them out in a sequence.

Take Joseph Pilates' advice: "Make a close study of each exercise and do not attempt any other exercise until you have mastered the current one" (Joseph Pilates, *Return to Life Through Contrology*).

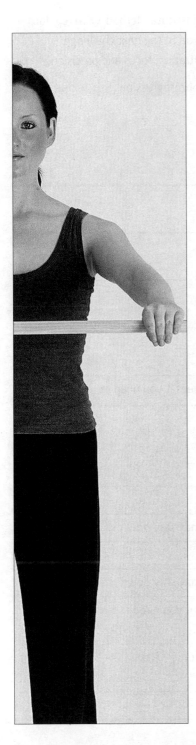

LEVEL 1

This is where you would start if you are unfamiliar with Pilates in general or the Pilates Institute Method. Even if you have some Pilates experience, it is always a good idea to re-visit the basics and reinforce the Pilates principles.

LEVEL 2

Now you are familiar with the introduction you are ready to start working a little harder – but don't forget the quality, precision and control of the movements.

LEVEL 3

This is when you are very confident with the exercises and can remember combinations, allowing you to create a more flowing session.

ROUTINE

Each workout begins with a preparation phase. Take this time to focus on the set up, the neutral spine alignment, the gentle engagement of the deep abdominals and the lateral breathing technique.

Finish each session with a few minutes of contemplation, noticing your breath and body alignment. Take a few extra minutes out to enjoy the feeling of wellbeing that the time you have given to yourself creates.

LEVEL 1 Option 1

These suggested programmes will help to introduce you to the Pilates Institute Method. With regular practice you will build a strong foundation that will allow you to move on to the next challenge. Consider the principles of the technique particularly, breathing, concentration, focus and precision.

Page	Exercise	Focus	Repetitions	Modification/progression

PREPARATION – SET UP

Page	Exercise	Focus	Repetitions	Modification/progression
34	Neutral Spine practice	Awareness	1 minute	
36	Engagement practice	Awareness	1 minute	
38	Breathing practice	Awareness	1 minute	
44	Arm Circles	Releasing Shoulders	5 in each direction	
46	Supported Side Bends	Lengthening	3 each side	
49	Roll Down	Mobility	3–5	Hand on knees if you need to

WORKOUT

Page	Exercise	Focus	Repetitions	Modification/progression
74	Hundred	Strength	5 breaths each leg x 2	
82	Single Leg Stretch	Strength	5 each leg	
88	Side Kick (1 side)	Strength	5–10 reps	Lower leg may stay down
92	Swimming	Strength	5 each leg/arm	
88	Side Kick (2nd side)	Strength	5–10 reps	Lower leg may stay down
98	Spine Twist	Mobility	5 each side alternating	Bend knees if you need to
84	Double Leg Stretch Modified	Mobility of shoulders	5-10 reps	Arm circles only
96	Shoulder Bridge	Mobility	5-10 reps	

LEVEL 1 Option 2

Page	Exercise	Focus	Repetitions	Modification/progression

WARM UP – SET UP

Page	Exercise	Focus	Repetitions	Modification/progression
34	Neutral Spine practice	Awareness		
36	Engagement practice	Awareness		
38	Breathing practice	Awareness		
45	Overhead Raise	Length	3–5 reps	

WORKOUT

Page	Exercise	Focus	Repetitions	Modification/progression
72	Push Up	Strength	3–5 reps	Bend knees as you roll down
74	Hundred	Strength	5 breaths each leg x2	
78	One Leg Circle	Mobility	5 each direction	Use hand on knee for support if necessary
88	Side Kick (1 side)	Strength	5–10 reps	Lower leg may stay down
86	Swan Dive	Mobility	3–5 reps	Turn toes in to release glutes
88	Side Kick (2nd Side)	Strength	5–10 reps	Lower leg may stay down
76	Roll Up	Strength	5–10 reps	Bend knees
82	Single Leg Stretch	Strength	5 each leg	

LEVEL 2   Option 1

Now you are familiar with the basic set up you can concentrate on working in a more challenging way. Concentration, Focus and Precision are the principles we are still working with – performing the movements with the best quality is your aim.

Page	Exercise	Focus	Repetitions	Modification/progression

WARM UP

Page	Exercise	Focus	Repetitions	Modification/progression
43	Set up Stance	Awareness	1–2 minutes	
44	Arm circles	Mobility	5–10 in each direction	
45	Overhead Raise	Mobility	5–10 reps	
61	Neck Stretch	Lengthening	3 each side	
61	Neck Rotations	Mobility	3 each side	
49	Roll Down	Mobility	5 reps	Bend knees and support with hand on thighs if hamstrings short

WORKOUT

Page	Exercise	Focus	Repetitions	Modification/progression
72	Push Up	Strength	5–8 reps	Option to walk hands further forward
86	Swan Dive	Mobility	5–8 reps	Turn toes in to release glutes
88	Side Kick (1 side)	Strength	10 reps	Try to keep lower leg lifted
96	Shoulder Bridge	Mobility	5–8 reps	
88	Side Kick (2nd side)	Strength	10 reps	Try to keep lower leg lifted
78	One Leg Circle	Mobility	5 in each direction	Try to take hand away from knee
94	Side Bend (1 side)	Strength	5 each side	
90	Scissors	Strength	5 each leg	
94	Side Bend (2nd side)	Strength	5 each side	
76	Roll Up	Strength	5–8 reps	

LEVEL 2 Option 2

Page	Exercise	Focus	Repetitions	Modification/progression

WARM UP

Page	Exercise	Focus	Repetitions	Modification/progression
43	Set Up Stance	Awareness	1–2 minutes	
44	Arm Circles	Mobility	5–10 reps	
61	Neck Stretch	Length	3 each side	
61	Neck Rotations	Mobility	3 each side	
46	Supported Side Bend	Length	3–5 each side	
49	Roll Down	Mobility	3 reps	Bend knees if necessary
50	Roll Down & Back Extension	Mobility	3 reps	Bend knees if necessary

WORKOUT

Page	Exercise	Focus	Repetitions	Modification/progression
92	Swimming	Strength	5 alternate arms 5 alternate legs	
85	Swan Dive	Mobility	5–8 reps	Turn toes in to release glutes
88	Side Kick (1 side)	Strength	10 reps	
74	Hundred	Strength		5–8 breathes each leg
88	Side Kick (2nd side)	Strength	10 reps	
98	Spine Twist	Mobility	5–8 each side alternating	
78	One Leg Circle	Mobility	5–8 in each direction	
96	Shoulder Bridge	Mobility	5–8 reps	
84	Double Leg Stretch Modified	Strength & mobility	5–8 reps	Circles arms back: hold single leg at right angle

LEVEL 3 Option 1

Before starting on the level 3 programmes, ensure that you are very clear about your understanding of the technique. These options are designed to challenge your strength and mobility. With your regular practice you will be confident about some of the movements without referring to the charts, so you can focus on the flowing movement that is so important to the Pilates technique. Do your best to move smoothly from one exercise to the next. This will help you create a full body movement programme that is the ultimate intention of the programme.

Page	Exercise	Focus	Repetitions	Modification/progression

WARM UP

Page	Exercise	Focus	Repetitions	Modification/progression
43	Set Up Stance	Awareness	1–2 minutes	
44	Arm Circles	Mobility	10 in each direction	Alternate the arms
45	Overhead Raise	Shoulder Stability	10 reps	Reduce reps if shoulders tire
46	Overhead Side Bend	Length & shoulder stability	5 each side	Use Supported Side Bend if you have low back issues
47	Roll Downs	Mobility	5 reps	Bend knees if necessary
50	Roll Downs & Extensions	Mobility	3–5 reps	Bend knees if necessary

WORKOUT

Page	Exercise	Focus	Repetitions	Modification/progression
74	Hundred	Strength	Up to 20 breaths each leg	Option to lift both legs
96	Shoulder Bridge	Mobility	10 reps	
78	One Leg Circle	Mobility	5–10 in each direction	Option to begin straightening the moving leg
88	Side Kick (1 side)	Strength	10 reps	Attempt to keep both legs lifted

Page	Exercise	Focus	Repetitions	Modification/progression
90	Scissors	Strength	5–10 reps each leg	Option to lengthen the moving leg or alternate the legs from the bottom of the movement
88	Side Kick (2nd side)	Strength	10 reps	Attempt to keep both legs lifted
100	Leg Pull Prone	Strength	Up to 20 breaths	
76	Roll Up	Strength	5–10 reps	Option for progression
94	Side Bend (1 side)	Strength	5–10 reps	
82	Single Leg Stretch	Strength	10 each leg alternating	Option to bring working leg to a right angle Both legs lifted
82	Side Bend (2nd side)	Strength	5–10 reps	
80	Rolling Like a Ball	Mobility	5–10 reps	Do not roll onto your neck Place hands on shins
72	Push Up	Strength & mobility	8 reps	Walk hands further out

LEVEL 3 Option 2

Page	Exercise	Focus	Repetitions	Modification/progression

WARM UP

	As option 1	Awareness	5–10 minutes	

WORK OUT

Page	Exercise	Focus	Repetitions	Modification/progression
74	Hundred both legs	Strength	Up to 20 breaths	Replace one leg if you lose neutral alignment
76	Roll Up	Strength	8–10 reps	With progression
98	Spine Twist	Mobility	10 reps alternating sides	
88	Side Kick (1 side)	Strength	10 reps	Both legs lifted
94	Side Bend (1 side)	Strength	5–10 reps	
96	Shoulder Bridge	Mobility	10 reps	
88	Side Kick (2nd Side)	Strength	10 reps	Both legs lifted
94	Side Bend (2nd side)	Strength	5–10 reps	
90	Scissors	Strength	10 reps each leg	Option to begin straightening moving leg or alternating legs from the bottom of the movement
82	Single Leg Stretch	Strength	10 reps each leg alternating	Option to bring working leg to a right angle Lift both legs
80	Rolling Like a Ball	Mobility	10 reps	Do not roll onto your neck Place hands on shins
100	Leg Pull Prone	Strength	Up to 20 breaths	
72	Push Up	Strength & mobility	5–8 reps	Walk hands further out

GLOSSARY

Abdominals The muscles layered across the midriff that lie across each other at various angles. There are four layers: the rectus abdominis, internal and external obliques and the transversus abdominis.

Alignment How your body is positioned in relation to gravity and the base of support.

Cervical Spine Portion of the spine contained in the neck – consisting of 7 vertebrae.

Coordination An organised working together of muscles aimed at bringing about purposeful movement.

Contrology The name that Joseph Pilates gave to his corrective method of exercise.

Flex To bend.

Imprinting Gently pressing the spine into the mat, tilting the pelvis backwards.

Ligaments Fibrous structures connecting bone to bone that provide support while allowing flexibility and movement.

Powerhouse The name Joseph Pilates gave to the abdominal area between the ribs and hips. It is from this "Powerhouse" that all Pilates movements start to help support and stabilise the lower back.

Prone Lying face down.

Repertoire The collection of movements that make up the Pilates Institute programmes.

Soften Knees holding the knees relaxed and slightly bent.

Shoulder Girdle The flesh and muscles connected with the shoulder joint and upper back.

Stack the Shoulders Place the shoulder one on top of the other (side lying).

Stance The attitude or position of a standing person.

Supine Lying on the back.

Vertebra One of the bony segments that make up the spinal column.

Visualisation Use of mental imagery to assist in the accomplishment of physical tasks, an important element of the Pilates technique to help with focus and concentration of the quality and performance of the movements.

Index

Acknowledgements

We would like to thank Scott Smith for his guidance in our early days, and our Project Management team for their continuous support

All photos copyright © Pilates Institute except: front cover top and middle, pages 7, 12, 13, 30 & 32 – Getty Images; page 5 – Mary Evans Picture Library; page 17 bottom right – Photodisk